Marc "Animal" MacYoung

Taking
It to the
Street

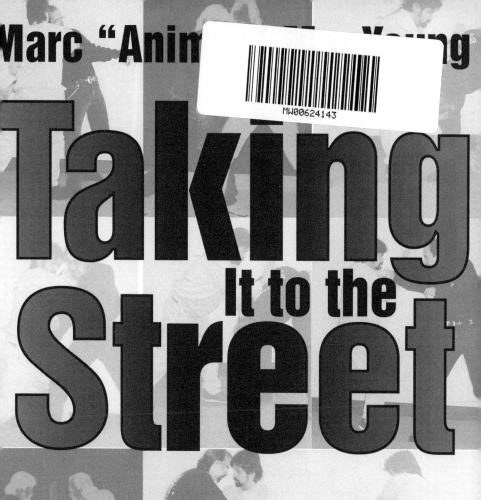

Making Your Martial Art
Street Effective

PALADIN PRESS · BOULDER, COLORADO

Also by Marc "Animal" MacYoung:

Cheap Shots, Ambushes, and Other Lessons
Down But Not Out (video)
Fists, Wits, and a Wicked Right
Floor Fighting
Knives, Knife Fighting, and Related Hassles
Pool Cues, Beer Bottles, & Baseball Bats
Safe in the City
Street E&E
Surviving a Street Knife Fight (video)
Violence, Blunders, and Fractured Jaws
Winning a Street Knife Fight (video)

Taking It to the Street: Making Your Martial Art Street Effective
by Marc "Animal" MacYoung

Copyright © 1999 by by Marc "Animal" MacYoung

ISBN 1-58160-050-X
Printed in the United States of America

Published by Paladin Press, a division of
Paladin Enterprises, Inc., P.O. Box 1307,
Boulder, Colorado 80306, USA.
(303) 443-7250

Direct inquires and/or orders to the above address.

Illustrations by Marc MacYoung
Visit Animal's Web site at www.diac.com/~dgordon

Visit Paladin's Web site at www.paladin-press.com

co~~TABLE OF~~ntents

Introduction

The difference between theory and practice
is in theory, there is no difference.

—An experienced engineer

In the movie *Platoon*, several guys fresh out of boot camp have just arrived in Vietnam and are about to go out on their first patrol. Although the movie doesn't show it, you can assume these kids have all the confidence of someone who doesn't have the faintest clue what's about to happen. (Sorry guys, but I've met young bucks straight out of boot camp before.)

Elias, the sergeant who will be leading the patrol, comes up to them with a look on his face like he's on his way to clean the latrines. He begins to strip off various parts of their gear with bored contempt, casually throwing away items and readjusting their webbing. The new guys are shocked and confused as this scruffy individual discards things that they were told in training were of vital importance for survival in the jungles of Vietnam. Elias, having crawled through Vietnamese jungles filled with people trying to shoot him, clearly indicates his opinion of what these kids were taught as "vital" for survival.

This scene is the first real indication to these kids that they aren't in Kansas anymore, and maybe things out here aren't quite like they were told back in boot camp.

Is Elias doing this to be cruel? Is he doing it to promote his as the ultimate way of doing things? To make lots of money by selling his secret fighting style to newcomers? No. It has nothing to do with ego, pride, or making money. It has everything to do with staying alive in a hostile environment. This isn't boot camp anymore—this is the real thing. And if you don't get the hang of what is going on, you're dead.

What these kids were trained for thousands of miles away isn't what is happening in the jungle war. Does this mean their training is useless? Some of it is. Some of it isn't. It's like that old business quip, "Half of my money in advertising is wasted. Problem is I don't know which half." The same can be said of your martial arts training. Figuring out which half is useless in a street fight is a bear. Unless you have an Elias to help you before you go out, the only way you're going to learn is in the middle of a firefight. Problem is, you may not survive the lesson. Trust me, they're not going to stop attacking when you say, "Hold on a minute, I have to figure out how to beat you."

Like the grunts in the field, if you want to survive the real thing, you're going to have to take your martial arts training and FIELDSTRIP! That means drop about half of what you know faster than a prom dress at 2 A.M. Then open your eyes and start learning all the stuff they didn't tell you about in school. That means looking at a situation and closely examining what you need to do with your martial arts training to make it work. I don't mean making it work in the dojo (we already know it does that), I mean making it work in the streets. In doing so, you must discard elements not directly related to effectively stopping an attack, or even worse, elements that would work directly against your survival. Believe me these elements are there.

ANIMAL'S IMPORTANT SAFETY TIP

- A blind spot is, by definition, not only a place that you can't see, but one that you don't know you can't see!

It isn't until you look at your skills from a different perspective that you begin to see holes and weaknesses. What looks like a solid defense from your point of view may have serious holes in it from another point of view. Unfortunately, that other point of view belongs to your attacker. It's not going to be until he's coming at you through them that you're going to find out about them holes—and by that time it's kinda late.

Throughout this book I'm going to be addressing a lot of those holes. I've been out there—in dark alleys, parking lots, honky tonks, and biker bars—and I've seen what works and what fails in the real thing.[1] When I tell you about a hole, take a look at it from several directions. Walk around it, look at it, kick it a few times, and experiment with it. Look for solutions inside your training and from other training sources. Get as many answers as you can. See what other people have to say about such a problem. But first and foremost, QUESTION YOUR TRAINING!

I know I speak blasphemy here against traditional martial arts, and I want you to know that, too. You're hearing bona fide, certified, out-and-out-heresy here. However, let me ask you something. It's the same decision those guys were facing in the jungle and the one you'll be facing in a dark alley.

The question is, what's more important—doing what you were trained to do or staying alive?

I am deadly serious about the importance of answering that question before you even consider using your training for self-defense. There are people who say, "Yeah, right. That's so obvious it's stupid." And then they turn around and go right back to exactly what they were doing. This is because THEY DON'T BELIEVE THAT THEY COULD BE KILLED OR INJURED DURING A REAL FIGHT!

That's bull! You can be. I am not talking about some hypothetical situation that you think you're trained for because you danced around the tournament ring a few times. I'm talking about getting your brains blown into a fine pink mist or sitting on a curb in shock as your bodily fluids leak out of a brand new hole. People who use violence to get their way hurt and kill others all the time. It's not a game out there. That guy coming at you out of the shadows with a weapon isn't playing. He will hurt you. And the odds are he's going to come at you in a totally different way than you were trained to handle. Surviving such an ugly event is exactly what this book addresses.

Answering this question is also important because it requires you to commit the worst heresy of them all—think for yourself, question doctrine, and, if necessary, break doctrine. If you don't think this a sore spot, you haven't been watching black-belt level politics at your school. Let me say right now, I am not here to disrespect your instructor, your style, or what you have worked so hard to achieve. But questioning what you have been taught is critical in order to fully understand what you know and what you don't know.

The *Tao te Ching* says, "Profit comes from what is there, usefulness comes from what is not there." The wheel is nice, but it's that empty space called the hub in the middle that makes it useful. The same can be said about your martial arts style. While you may have really profited from knowing your style, much of its usefulness for self-defense comes from knowing where it *doesn't* work! People who think their art is all encompassing often don't retreat from situations that are not favorable. This is real important since seldom will someone attack you in an area that is favorable to you. Most often, it will be under circumstances favorable to him. Otherwise, he wouldn't be attacking!

Let me give you a real basic idea of what I'm talking about. Environment is something that doesn't mean much in the dojo, but is of critical import in the real thing. Looking at the environmental limitations of your style is vital. For example, how would your style do on ice? What about in a cramped area, such as between two cars? Ever trained in the dark? How about on stairs? Uneven footing? Then come size and range issues. How would you fare against someone twice your size? How do you handle a sudden head-down-arms-spread-bull-like rush? What do you do against a small guy who wants to shimmy up your leg and bite your kneecap off? Ever trained against someone who doesn't overcommit himself to a punch? Boxers are nasty. Oh, yeah, let's not forget weapons! These elements (and many others) are part of real-life scenarios. Have you trained for them? Finding yourself fighting for your life in these circumstances is a harsh way to learn your style's limits.

By asking these questions, you don't subtract

from the art—you learn. There is nothing wrong with asking, "Where won't this work?" I've repeatedly said that different martial arts styles were designed to work in different environments. Within a specific environment, they are absolutely devastating (like wing chun in cramped quarters or tae kwon do in open areas), but take them out of those areas and you have problems. The same can be asked about your training. Where doesn't it work? And why?

Aside from environmental considerations, over the years a whole lot of ineffective moves have crept into styles courtesy of sports emphasis. While sports fighting is not bad in and of itself, recognizing the difference between sport and self-defense is muy importanto. The big difference is that there are rules in tournaments. This affects—in a major way—how you fight.

It's not fun to think of it, but those tournament moves are exactly what an experienced fighter will turn against you. Sports fighters hit for points and psychological damage. A streetfighter doesn't care about causing psychological damage; every blow he throws is for the sole purpose of causing physical damage. If it doesn't do that, he doesn't bother throwing it. You can bet he's real happy to go up against someone who doesn't share his philosophy. (By the way, if someone doesn't back off when you tell him you're a black belt, it's a pretty sure bet you're up against an experienced brawler. You done treed yourself a bad one there, Billy Bob). You can also bet he isn't interested in causing cumulative damage that will manifest in later rounds. He wants to drop the whole enchilada on you now.

Traditional moves are another source of martial arts techniques that often don't work on the street. These once made sense, but they stayed around after the situation changed and have been passed on by rote. Again, not bad if you recognize them for what they are. Practically speaking, though, these moves have no application for the kind of conflict you'll find yourself in. For example, next time you need to take a mounted warrior off a horse, them flying sidekicks are just the thing. However, if you need to get someone off a motorcycle it's easier and faster just to clothesline the guy. This saves you all sorts of embarrassment about accidentally flying by your target because motorcycles move faster than horses. Of course, them overhead double-handed cross blocks are smoking for being attacked by a samurai with a sword. That happens to me ALL the time! How about you?

In order to effectively fieldstrip, we're going to approach the arts from a different perspective.

The first variation is that we are not going to just jump right into how to split heads. That comes later. There is a whole lot more going on during real fights than just crackin' someone's coconut. To quote Pogo: "We have met the enemy and he is us." Boy is that true in this business.

ANIMAL'S IMPORTANT SAFETY TIP

- Most people who lose a fight aren't defeated by their opponent, they defeat themselves.

That puts a totally different spin on the subject, doesn't it? Before you can hope to defeat someone, you have to make sure you don't shoot yourself in the foot. The only way to do that is to know what is going on inside of you so you don't trip over yourself. While some of what I talk about may sound kind of spacey, let me tell you from having actually been there—these issues can spell the difference between life and death. Your choice, though. If you're impatient, the "les jes bash 'im onna head" stuff of Br'er Bear fu starts around Chapter 5. But if you're interested in living long enough to lie to your grandkids, you might want to muddle through the earlier chapters.

The second variation is that our approach to self-defense will emphasize principles rather than techniques. The difference is simple: THINKING. I will tell you right now that the best fighters I have ever met have all been principles fighters. It is their understanding of principles and their ability to immediately apply them that makes them the sort of people Hollywood makes movies about.

The difference between principles and techniques is the same as that between strategy and tactics in military applications. Strategy is the overview—call it the general plan, if you will. Tactics are how you manifest that strategy in a particular place. You tailor your tactics to fit the circumstances. In this case, you have to be the military leader. You have to take the strategy (principles) and come up with the tactics (techniques) that will ensure your command's success as they go through unfamiliar territories with hostiles around. If you figure out how the principle works, you will automatically know the best technique to use at the moment.

This issue of techniques vs. principles has also begun to cross over to teaching. I prefer to teach principles and show you how to apply them. (I am not alone in this new approach. We're still a minority, but our numbers are growing.) What most old-style instructors call the basics, I call tools. What I call basics are the fundamental principles on how things work. Believe me, there is a huge difference between their basics and my fundamental principles.

Let me give you an example of the difference.

Let's say you want to learn plumbing. Most people will teach you the basics first—things like this is a pipe wrench, these are the various sizes of pipes, etc. You can spend a lot of time learning these. Yet, when it is all said and done, you still won't know how to fix a toilet. You'll know the names of the tools and what they are for, but you won't know how to use them or how to diagnose a problem. That comes from learning tools as basics.

The way I work is that I start with a fundamental principle like, "Water flows downhill—if that ain't happening, something is stopping it." Everything we do to fix the problem will pretty much relate to getting that principle back on line. This includes examining the toilet to find at what point the water stops flowing downhill and throwing in what you need to know about the specific tools for the job. The main focus, however, is and always has been fixing the toilet. By knowing the principle from the start, you have a better chance of achieving that goal.

Most often, martial arts training is like learning plumbing the old-fashioned way. It gives you the basic tools, but it doesn't really give you the principles on how to use them to fix a real-life problem. Consider this with regard to techniques you learn by rote. Under fixed circumstances I tell you to do this, you do it, you learn it. After doing it long enough, you begin to quickly and unconsciously apply this knowledge in sparring matches. You see the opportunity and react. Somehow it's sunk to a deeper level where, under specific circumstances, you can use it automatically. Granted, it has taken years of practice, but you've got a general idea of how it works.

If you focus only on techniques, the things you've learned may never sink in to that deeper level where you instinctively grasp the concepts involved rather than just react to certain stimuli. Why is this important? Because it's only when you understand the fundamental principles that you can effectively react no matter what is happening. Now instead of waiting for a specific set of circumstances (which may never come) to apply a particular technique, you can create a technique that works at that moment.

Instead of asking you to devote years to rote training on techniques, hoping that you'll unconsciously grasp the principles, I'm going to flop those principles on the table like a big dead fish and hand you a knife. We're going to gut that sucker right off. You'll learn by doing as we go.

Bruce Lee said of fighting, "It's always changing." You can know 10,000 techniques and in the real thing discover that you only needed to know one—a different one.

However, by looking at this subject from the viewpoint of principles, you will begin to see that what at first seemed like a whirl of countless differences is actually just simple variations on some very basic themes.

A single principle can spawn thousands of techniques—all of which will work under different circumstances. Don't focus on what is different in every situation; instead learn to see what remains constant! If you understand the principle, you can look at a situation and say, "Nope, that technique won't work, but this one will. BOOM! Yep, it worked."

If you don't have this deeper understanding, it's always going to be a "whadda I do?! whadda I do?!" situation where you are throwing all sorts of stuff, hoping something is going to work. When you know the principle, it's just a matter of making it manifest in any situation.

I'll give you an important hint right now, one

that will help you learn faster whatever style you study. As you now know, techniques are manifestations of principles. A very important function of principles is that they help you to categorize information. By learning how to think along the lines of principles, you will create a mental filing system that will cut your learning time in half. Instead of learning 27 different kicks one at a time, you'll learn there are four types of kicks. Every kick you learn gets tossed into one of these categories. You don't have to learn 27 kicks from scratch, as every kick is just a variation on a basic theme.

If you drive a car, you already do this kind of thinking. It's taken you years, but now you do it quickly, easily, and unconsciously. You drive, something changes, and you adjust what you're doing accordingly. A rule as simple as "for every 10 mph, keep a car length between you and the car in front of you" can result in a wide variety of actions, such as changing lanes, speeding up, or braking. It's an ongoing process, depending on what is happening one minute to the next. Like I said, you do this kind of thinking already. You just don't know that's what you've been doing. What I am doing is just bringing it to your attention.

Quite often after I've done a move, people come up to me and ask, "Where did you study judo/jujutsu/aikido, etc.?" When I tell them I have no formal training in those arts, they are amazed and usually say, "But that was a perfect (fill in the blank) technique." It wasn't, at least not to me.

Whatever I did was just the best way to apply a principle at that moment. Their style has a name for it, and they had to train long and hard to be able to do that particular move. Me, I just did what I knew would work at the moment. Which one is really simpler?

If you take these concepts and apply them in tournaments and sparring matches before you try them out on the street, you'll see that they really do work. Fiddle around with them in the safety of the dojo and with people you trust. Not only will they help you in winning your sparring matches (and maybe a tournament or two), but more importantly you'll learn how they work and to trust in their effectiveness. Incidentally, later on I describe what real fights are like, so you might also want to practice them under safer circumstances with a sparring partner coming at you like the real thing.

---

[1] If you would like a rundown on my "street" qualifications, read Appendix A.

CHAPTER 1

The Four Focuses of the Martial Arts (or "We Be Here")

....

Do you know the actual problem, or are you guessing?

—Tony J.

In my opinion, many people who write books about making martial arts street effective make two major mistakes. The first is they often spend way too much time telling people how useless the traditional martial arts are. The second is they tell you to become kung fu killers. Let's take them one at a time.

The first is a real turnoff. These guys bag on everything you've learned. They drone endlessly on how tournaments encourage bad habits, how martial arts don't work in the street, how the arrogance and cockiness of many martial artists will get them hurt when they meet someone dedicated to hurting them, how ineffective the Westernized or business martial art schools are, how they're just belt factories, blah, blah, blah, blah, etc., etc. . . . Obviously, while these guys may have some seriously valid points, they have gone to the Charging Rhino School of Tact and Social Graces.

As I once told a woman who was flipping out on me about a screw-up by one of my bouncers, "Lady, you're right, but you're being so obnoxious that I don't care."[1] This is exactly what these clowns are doing. The validity of their points is lost behind how they're presenting them. Nobody likes being told that what they worked long and hard at is useless. This is especially true if you've been doing it in good faith that it would work out on the streets.

By coming out and saying that other people's styles are useless, these critics are being short-sighted, disrespectful, and rude. They also are over-looking a major issue. There are focuses to the martial arts other than just cracking skulls and breaking bones. And I'll bet dollars to doughnuts that it's another focus that you regularly deal with in your martial arts.

In essence, they are saying that their focus on the martial arts is right and everyone else's is wrong. Unfortunately, on the subject of stepping out of bounds, the door swings both ways. There *are* a lot of instructors out there who are giving these guys legitimate axes to grind about what the martial arts teach as self-defense. What these instructors are doing is taking their focus and trying to pass it off as street-effective self-defense.

What do I mean by focus? Simply stated, in the Western world there are four major focuses in the martial arts.

1. The self-defense/combat application is pretty much only concerned with crunching someone's head. It's how to kill or hurt an opponent so badly that he is no longer a threat. It can also mean professional use of force for police, hospi-

tal staff, security, or anyone else whose job it is to head toward trouble instead of away from it. Generally, these moves aren't pretty, flashy, or complicated—just brutally effective.

2. The physical art/tradition/discipline (both physical and mental) is what most schools really teach. They're teaching a physical art form or a tradition that requires great dedication, self-discipline, and focus to achieve. I have seen kids bloom in the martial arts, and I've seen the benefits spread through their lives in everything from schoolwork and social skills to improved home life.[2] Most people who get into the martial arts get into this aspect, and it helps them improve their lives through both physical and mental work.

3. The spiritual development/health aspect is incredible. Although on the surface it looks woo-woo, I've seen enough to know that something very real is going on. I have met people who follow the martial arts as a spiritual path, and they are amazing. I also remember seeing a photo of an old Chinese man who was 80 years if he was a day standing there relaxed and smiling . . . on one foot . . . hand up in the air . . . his body held horizontal . . . one foot off the ground. I was 30 at the time, and there was no way I could have managed that stance. Yet here is a guy with 50 years on me doing it and smiling. Tell me this isn't powerful stuff for your health!

4. The sports aspect is a blast. It's great for channeling young aggressive energy. And to be good at it calls for some serious dedication and hard work. It's something you can personally get involved with, and it is fun. It's a great confidence builder, and it's also loads of fun to watch.

Each of these focuses represents a very real and valid reason to study the martial arts. No one way is more valid or more important than any other way, regardless of what a particular proponent of one focus may tell you. Different styles, schools, and teachers tend to dwell on different focuses. On top of that, we tend to gravitate toward what focus is most important to us.

The focus you study says hundreds of things about you. It affects how you're trained, what you think about the art, what moves you do, how you move, etc. Each focus has different benefits, strengths, drawbacks, and teachings. Each focus has its own goals, and way it is taught is tailored to reach those goals.

While a particular martial art style can lean heavily toward a particular focus, it's usually the teacher who takes it the rest of the way. These teachers tend to attract people who want or need that same focus.[3] It's kind of like a critter evolving to a specific environment.

If a particular focus doesn't fit your needs, that doesn't mean it's useless or less effective than your chosen focus. It just means it's different. It took me years to realize this. When I was younger, I had total contempt for tradition- and sports-focused arts. Simply stated, they didn't serve my needs. I was busy trying to keep from getting my brains blown out, and these guys were going on about kata, self-discipline, and winning tournaments. "Uhhhhh, I don't think this what I need, guys." It wasn't my focus. Naturally, I left those schools for places that better suited my needs. Unfortunately, back then I was ticked off because I felt that those guys had lied to me.

To tell the truth, some *had* consciously lied to me, trying to peddle what they had as self-defense (yeah, right). Others had honestly offered what they thought would work or had tried to offer what they thought I needed. In all cases, though, what they did was put forth a different focus to solve what was to them a theoretical problem. The guy coming at them in the dojo was a padded, protected player looking to win a tournament, while the guy coming at me on the street swinging a car jack had slightly different intentions. I couldn't afford to spend years learning how to stop that sort of thing. Nor could I afford the sports mentality of, "I can soak up a few blows before I kick his butt." Not when there were weapons and large numbers of attackers involved.

Unfortunately, this is still happening. I hear from countless people who are facing this same problem. They get frustrated when they don't get what they want out of a particular school or teacher. They're looking for the first focus, and what they're getting is the same thing I went through.

I have nearly 30 years experience in a wide variety of martial arts and entirely too much real-time application. Yet, I can't claim to have mastered more than one focus. And I'm still learning stuff about my area of expertise. But as good as I am in one area, it doesn't translate into other areas. My mind-set is totally different.

For example, I am not a sports fighter. The idea that I *don't* have to cover something tender or that I *can't* rip it off my opponent because it's against the rules is totally foreign to me. A "no-no move" is unthinkable to me. If it's there, it's fair game. The idea of hitting, skipping back, and pausing so the ref can call a point is incomprehensible. Come to think of it, listening to a ref tell me to step off someone's face isn't really understandable to me either. (Doesn't he know how hard I worked to get there in the first place?) And while I'm on a soapbox, I've noticed that they get really upset when you pick up and use a chair in a tournament.

I will be the first to tell you I don't know other focuses. When I teach police and military, what I show them has no tradition, discipline, or spiritual application, and it definitely isn't a sport. It lands directly in the realm of focus No. 1: Get the job done. Do it fast and without injury to yourself. We don't have belts or levels. Our goal is you up, him down. How badly hurt he is depends on what job you're doing. This is my focus. It's definitely for high-risk situations and nothing else.[4]

As to the other focuses, I don't have a clue. Want to reach satori? Errr . . . um . . . take I-10 and turn left at Albuquerque? Live a long healthy life? Don't let her husband catch you together? I couldn't even begin to tell you how to win in a kata competition. I guarantee you, I'll get you kicked out of a tournament if you use what I teach. Tradition? Try Devil's Night in Detroit, that's about how much I know about that subject. Discipline? Isn't that where people run around in a lot of leather and do kinky things to each other? Basically, I know my focus very well, but I also know that I don't know others.

I will say right here and now that mastering all the aspects is nigh unto impossible. Maybe you can master two, but that's rare. I have met only one person of whom it could be said that he had mastered three. Here are some qualifiers to that statement, though: first, he was an 87-year-old; second, he was a grandmaster; third, he would have denied it; and fourth, he disapproved of the arts being used as sports—which kind of closed that focus down. His main focuses were spirit/health and tradition/discipline, and that's what he taught![5]

There is no ultimate martial art or fighting style. That's because there is no one ultimate focus of the martial arts. Each of us seeks the focus that is right for us. What is best for you won't be what is best for me or for someone else. Respect each focus for what it is and its inherent value. Respect a person for the work he/she has put into that focus and the dedication it took to get there.

Having said that, however, let me point out something real important. Problems occur when someone oversteps the boundaries of his focus and tries to pass it off as another. For example, I get real persnickity about someone who teaches sport karate calling it self-defense to attract students. It's not that such people don't know their focus, but that they are trying to claim mastery in a focus they don't know![6]

This is what I am referring to with the question, "Do you know the actual problem or are you just guessing?" Most people who claim to teach self-defense don't know what a real attack is like. Many have never been in a fight in their lives, while others haven't been in one since high school. I will tell you right now that the three dudes stepping out of the shadows aren't interested in a mano-a-mano high school fight.

I am as serious as a heart attack with what I am about to say here. Under these circumstances, complicated, fantasyland self-defense moves are dangerous to you, the student. Odds are those guys stepping out of the shadows have weapons, too. This here ain't no tournament, Sport. What you've learned for tournament fighting isn't going to work here. Under these circumstances, knowing which 50 percent of what you know is useless becomes real important.

Approaching the focus of self-defense like it's a tournament is like believing you can pogo stick through a mine field. Until you try, you may think

you can get away with it. But when you find yourself in the middle of the real thing, the results won't
be pleasant. I don't care if it's point sparring or
hardcore full-contact sport fighting you do. The real
thing is a different ballgame. The problem is that
every year martial art schools hand out more and
more pogo sticks . . . excuse me, black belts. Many
of those black belts, like those kids in *Platoon*, think
they know what they're doing! I mean, after all,
isn't this what they were trained for?

No, this is the jungle, and out here we have to
fieldstrip.

This issue of different focuses is why it is so critical for you to objectively look at and dissect any
technique that your instructor tells you is a "self-
defense" move. It's like a kali guy bragging that he's
a knife fighter without ever having been in a knife
fight. Whether it's intentional lying or self-delusion,
it just ain't so![7] You can spend a lot of time learning
what he thinks is self-defense. Problem is, it will be
your blood if you ever have to use it in a real situation. Learn it for what it is, but don't expect it to
work in the real thing.

In order for your martial art to be effective in a
real situation, you have to strip it down. You have to
do this to see what can work in a totally different
set of circumstances. The fact that most people will
never find themselves in such a situation makes it
hard to winnow the wheat from the chaff. In order
to fieldstrip, you need to know two things: First,
you have to be aware of how you were trained. In
other words, know what your current focus is. You
can't get someplace else if you don't know where
you are starting from. Second, before you get there
you must learn what the conditions are in the new
place. I'll cover a lot of these in the next few chapters. Once you have a general idea you can begin to

look at techniques from the standpoint of, "would it work under these conditions?"

From a student's standpoint, it is not disrespectful to know and accept the strengths and limitations of your teacher's skills and focus. In fact, I also want you to do the same with what I'm telling you. You're not going to hurt my little duck feelings if you decide to do something different than what I recommend. It's your butt that's on the line here, not his, not mine. You do what works for you. Think for yourself, and always remember with any information, regardless of its source, "Check, double check, and check again."

Now we move on to the second mistake most people who write these kinds of books make: they tell you to become kung fu killers—total animals who'd just as soon bite the throat out of someone as look at him. OK plan . . . if you like taking showers with heavily tattooed guys named "Chester the Molester." If not, let's think about that idea for a second. The problem with that attitude is, simply, we live in a society with laws about the reasonable use of force. Add to that we have people called police who enforce those laws. Going ballistic on someone is NOT a good way to avoid spending lots of time and money learning the intricacies of our legal system.

ANIMAL'S IMPORTANT SAFETY TIP

- The cops tend to arrest the winner of the fight. They see him as the one in the wrong and who went overboard—because usually this is the case. In real fights the person who becomes violent first most often wins. Add to this that the person who becomes violent first usually is the main instigator. Do the math, winner = aggressor. That's how they look at it. Amazingly enough, 99 percent of the time they're right.

So you can see how easy it would be for the police to misinterpret your successfully defending yourself. Oh yeah, guess what? It's going to get more complicated when the guy who attacked you lies and says you started it—which he will do![8] Trust me on this one, I've been there, done that. If you Taz'ed out on the guy and started jumping up and down on his chest like these books say, his broken bones are going to give his lie credibility. You, not he, will be arrested or charged.

Peyton Quinn[9] told me of an incident in which he and his friend were coming out of a nightclub and got jumped by four guys swinging 2x4s. The guys had lain in ambush for them after a verbal confrontation inside. One of the attackers blindsided Peyton's friend, and he dropped with a cracked skull. Peyton pulled up the killer instinct and blitzkrieged the attackers. He then got his friend to the hospital in time to save his life. You can imagine that with a seriously wounded comrade, he didn't loiter around and kick these guys while they were down. However, Peyton was later sued by these very guys. Because they were hurt, they claimed *he* started the fight, and, because of that, he owed *them* damages! It took him thousands of dollars in lawyer and private investigator fees before he was cleared of any wrongdoing. Even though he was in the right, it cost him a lot of money and hardship.

Oh yeah, if you think that by being a fresh-faced nice person your innocence will be immediately obvious to the police, let me point out that entirely too many clean-cut, respectable people go out and buy drugs from exactly this kind of scum. This could have been a drug deal gone bad. Cops see that a lot.

If after defending yourself you stick around until the cops show up, you had better have a real good reason as to why you were there in the first place because it will get ugly.

That is the reality of what happens when you use that much touted "killer instinct" in our world. So while it can be important for your survival, it can and does cause a host of problems on its own. Those problems are in areas where you least expect them. It's not a game, it's not an ego thing, and it definitely isn't something you just turn on and off when you get bored playing with it. Tinkering around with the psyche on this level can have life-long repercussions, so consider well why you want to go there.

The other problem I have with this mentality is it assumes you're ready. That's to say you have spent years preparing yourself to be able to explode into total, vicious, bone-breaking violence at the drop of a hat. (Gee . . . with an attitude like that your social calendar must be booked. Let me guess, you get your dates at "Psychos R Us.") Or it assumes that you've had time to mentally prepare yourself, change clothes, square off, and are just waiting for the bell so you can come out of your corner swinging. If this were the case, you'd be in a sparring match instead of a fight.

Realistically, what this idea of the Ronco-Instamatic-kung-fu-killer doesn't cover is your minding your own business, walking to your car and thinking about something else, when suddenly someone steps out of a shadow with a weapon and nasty intentions. It's a big step from figuring out what you want for lunch to ripping someone's liver out (although it does tend to make the first problem moot). Nor does it cover if you're having a good time at a social gathering and all of sudden someone unexpectedly takes umbrage with the fact that you're breathing. Next thing you know, it went from a nice evening to someone jumping in your face. Believe it or not, the insta-werewolf routine is hard to do, even if you're arguing with someone. His taking a swing at times like this is a surprise! ("Hey! wait a minute! When did it go from verbal to physical?!")

This is how fights really happen. And to tell you the truth, they catch people off guard. I know a woman who is a 4th-degree black belt who was swung upon by a 19-year-old who had been giving her son problems. It was so unexpected that this woman—who had more than 10 years experience in martial arts—SAT DOWN in shock! Where she's from, when an adult gives a kid a piece of her mind, the kid isn't supposed to react that way! Well, someone forgot to tell the kid that. A decade of practice went out the window because she couldn't believe this kid chose an option she didn't expect.[10]

This is not to say books that try to teach the killer instinct are without merit. In fact, if you can keep from kissing the floor when the guy unexpectedly launches his attack they can be very useful for blasting out of ugly situations. However, that's not what *this* book is about. Understand, this book is not about how to kick ass. It's about how to keep your ass from getting kicked! Believe me that differentiation is no small matter. It's important to buy yourself enough time to get over the shock of being unexpectedly assaulted. This without getting your face pushed inside out! Remember who's saying that. If I can be surprised by a guy unexpectedly launching at me, so can you.

I'll let you in on a little secret—in the real thing not only does the other side hit back, but often they hit first. I've had my nose moved around my face a few times discovering this little truth. This tendency to unexpectedly blitzkrieg you is why focusing on preventing his attack from being successful comes before any other consideration. Trust me, it's nearly impossible to get over the shock of being attacked and organize a viable response while someone is tap dancing on your face.

I don't expect you to have the killer instinct, but I want you to be able to stay safe long enough to figure out what to do about being attacked—regardless of what he's doing. No matter how much training they have, most people get overwhelmed in those first few critical seconds. Think about it: How likely is it that you could successfully activate your training while someone is monkey-stomping you? All the training in the world won't do you a whit of good if you don't have a chance to use it. That means staying intact during a bushwhacking long enough to do something about it!

That's your first priority. Once you have that down, you can figure out the best thing to do to resolve the situation. Whether that means Taz'ing out on the guy and hitting him until he's flat or running at the speed of sound depends on the exact circumstances.

This is not to say that there are not times to go ballistic on folks. The tricky parts of doing it are figuring out if it's the right time and place to do so and shifting mental gears from your everyday way of thinking and getting to that place. Believe me, it's a long, hard jump to do quickly. Doing it is more difficult if someone is already whomping on you. And last but not least, there's dealing with the aftermath. Such issues as legalities, revenge seekers, and your own mental well-being last long after the fight is over.

Achieving this skill of surviving ambushes will give you time to regroup and decide what to do.

Consider that no matter what you decide to do, if he can't hit, you you can't hurt you! If he can't hurt you, he ain't gonna be winning is he?

Bringing up such reality breaks is why, in martial arts circles, I'm looked upon with the same regard as a noisome little troll who comes in sounding like Bobcat Goldthwaite, saying, "Excuse me . . . " They know when they see me coming, a monkey wrench is heading for their nice, neat little system. What can I say? I believe in peer review. I don't like junk science, and I don't like junk martial arts.

---

[1] Not the brightest or most tactful thing I could have said. She immediately ran to my boss. Fortunately, she flipped out on him, too. He much more tactfully told her essentially the same thing. Then he called me and gave me the "while it's true, that was a really stupid thing to say" lecture. Oops.

[2] It's also great for kids with Attention Deficit Disorder (ADD).

[3] I often say people come to the martial arts to learn self-defense but stay for other reasons. For the people who stay, whatever it is in that school, it's right for them. On the other hand, people who leave aren't getting what they wanted.

[4] Incidentally, I will be the first to admit that this is the most limited focus of the martial arts. While it is a necessary skill for certain professions and lifestyles, it has no real redeeming value within society. Having this talent will in no way help you raise a family, keep a job, improve your schoolwork, make you smooth with women, keep you healthy, or spiritually enlighten you. This focus is only good for an extremely limited set of circumstances.

[5] With this in mind, you can imagine what I think about 27-year-old self-proclaimed grandmasters of their own styles. I may not be the sharpest crayon in the box, but even I can figure out that something would be lacking from such a style in light of the four focuses.

[6] This often is caused by the guy's need to have students in

order to stay open. This is especially true when the instructor is making his living from the school. Unfortunately, as the moron—who looked me straight in the eye and said he'd never had a takedown not work—showed, a lot of the time it's from arrogance and lack of real experience.

[7] I regularly get kali, arnis, and even occasionally silat guys in my knife classes who say, "Whoa! This isn't like anything we know!" And that is true; much knife training is based not on your suddenly being ambushed (which is how it always seems to happen out there), but rather that it's going to be a "duel." (Got that term from Col. Rex Applegate. We were sitting around and he said most of what was being taught as knife fighting these days is dueling. I looked at him and said, "I'm going to steal that.")

[8] I'll give you a hint. The guy wants to win. He wants to walk away after having gotten the last lick in. If he can't do it physically, he's going to try to nail you in another way. That's why you can rely on him to lie.

[9] Author of *A Bouncer's Guide to Barroom Brawling* and *Real Fighting: Adrenaline Stress Conditioning through Scenario-Based Training*. Currently, Peyton lives just a few miles down the road from me in the highlands of Colorado. He runs Rocky Mountain Combat Applications Training, which is a scenario-based training system I recommend.

[10] The good news is that her reaction scared the kid enough that he split. He didn't keep on attacking. Realize that this was in a nice, quiet, Wonderbread kind of neighborhood where taking a poke at an adult is almost unheard of. Whereas there he was considered a total wildman, in my old neighborhood even the cheerleaders would have chased him down the street and kicked his butt for swinging on them.

CHAPTER 2

Let's Get the Rules Straight

*Fear can be your greatest enemy or
your best friend.*
*It can warm the belly and make you
feel alive*
or it can burn you up and destroy you.
—David Gemmell, *Waylander II*

WHAM!

The guy's fist crashing into my cheek told me that diplomacy definitely wasn't working. OK, I'd tried. His next punch was rudely interrupted by my counterpunch. I don't know if it was a wing chun punch, boxing, Shaolin, karate, kali, or a silat move. All I know is it got in his way. His didn't get through, but mine did. About two seconds later, slamming him into the ground was my subtle way of informing him his blitzkrieg had just run into a lightning rod. Ah well, the best laid schemes o' mice an' men gang aft a-gley, dude.

What is important to understand is that sometimes diplomacy works, sometimes it doesn't. In his case, diplomacy didn't work because he had decided that instead of talking, he could get what he wanted faster by being violent. Much to his dismay, he discovered that he really should have stuck with sweet reason. Even though he was willing to go there faster than I, I was better at being unreasonable. That was something he hadn't planned for when he decided to get froggy. Oops, STBY, Pal.[1]

In all honesty, it really didn't matter how tough I showed myself to be. This clown was a) so drunk and b) so wrapped up in what was going on in his head that he couldn't see it. This is a common problem with bozos who think they can beat Godzilla to death with their dicks. The only way they're going to know it's time to back off is when you slam them into the ground. What can I say? Stupid is as stupid does.

There are some situations that will NOT be resolved without fighting. In those cases, something is just wrong with the bozo's wiring. Nothing you do or say will stop the guy from moving on you. This is often the result of one or both of the issues I just mentioned—booze and internal garbage. They combine into a mind-set wherein the twit can't see anything beyond the inside of his own head, and that is what he is reacting to. Guys like this are dumb enough to swing on cops, so you can bet they're dumb enough to swing on you.

Realistically, though, violence is unavoidable in only about 10 percent of the situations you'll find yourself in. That means if you can find the right answer there is a 90-percent chance of negotiating your way out of trouble. So look at it this way, there is going to be a flat-out 10 percent of situations that will just go ballistic, no matter what you do or say. It is going to go sideways and there is nothing you can do about it.

Just because you don't have any control about whether it goes physical with that 10 percent doesn't mean you don't have any control about what happens after that point. Having dealt with way too many of these morons over the years, I have some good news for you. Most of them aren't that good at fighting. It's kind of like sex—just because they're willing to jump right in and go to town doesn't mean they're good at it. Most rely on mad-dog aggressiveness and swinging first to do all the work for them. They never learned to do anything else. When their Plan A fails, they're in a world of trouble because they don't have a Plan B. So despite their aggressiveness, these pudknockers are easy to deal with once you know how. The really good news is that what you're going to learn in this book is designed to work against this very sort of attack. So settle with the fact that it will occasionally go to hell in a hand basket, and, when it does, the only thing you can do is be better at it than the other guy.

Having said that, however, let's look at the other 90 percent. It is here, for good or bad, that you have real control. You can keep it from going physical, but it requires some work. The term 90 percent is somewhat misleading. It doesn't mean that every 9 out of 10 potential fights will end up without violence. It means 9 out of 10 conflicts CAN be resolved without violence. It's up to you to make it happen.

There are some people in this world who can make those 9-out-of-10 odds work. I've seen these people talk down situations that I was certain were 10-percenters. Then there are other people who just seem to be able to set off a situation. These jokers can take that 10 percent that goes bad and turn it into 100 percent. Fortunately, most of us land somewhere in the middle. It all boils down to how you handle people.

I will tell you right now that the stand-up-puff-up-your-chest-throw-your-arms-back-and-call-him-names response (all in hopes of letting him know how tough you are) is one of the best ways to guarantee a fight—as are any variations on that sort of move. But that is what most people think is the way to handle someone getting in your face. It is, in fact, the fastest way to disaster.

ANIMAL'S IMPORTANT SAFETY TIP

- The best way to avoid fights is not by being the baddest dude on the block, but knowing human nature.

Having a sense about your fellow man—how he thinks, how he acts, and what motivates him is the greatest skill you can ever have. It can save you all sorts of hassles, not only for avoiding fights, but for getting through life. In truth, the only thing that won't change in your life is the fact that you are surrounded by people. They will be with you from beginning to end. And that is why you should spend as much time as you can learning about how the silly buggers think and behave.

The more you know about how we as humans operate, the better your chances of getting your fights down to the 10 percent instead of 50/50—or worse—odds. Even better, you can go a long way toward avoiding trouble in the first place. Knowing human nature will do wonders for keeping you from getting thrown through walls by some pissed-off gorilla.[2]

On a more philosophical bent, violence and diplomacy are two halves of a whole. Each is more effective when backed by the other. Unfortunately, way too many people prefer one or the other. This brain-damaged philosophy also tends toward the Toys R Us version of whichever one a person picks.

In the Western world, intellectuals tend to go

into liver-quivering joy over the idea that "the pen is mightier than the sword." They are forgetting the first part *and* the qualifier of that sentence: "Under men entirely great . . ." (I dunno, maybe they think they automatically qualify.) The thing is, their weapons are words and that is where they want it to stay. I've noticed that many who use words as weapons have others to do the actual dirty work for them—whether it be another person, an agency, or legal action. They will sic someone else on you when their words don't work. It's kind of a glorified I'll-tell-mom-on-you attitude.[3]

Then there are those idiots who have learned that they can quickly get what they want by using violence. Since the depths of these people's intellect usually bottoms out like a puddle in a parking lot, they seldom see that this is a dead-end philosophy. If word gets out that you're a violent, unreasonable person, it's easier to just not deal with you. You'll get shuffled off into one of society's out-of-the-way "trash cans" (where such behavior is tolerated), and you'll be forgotten.[4] This is the social equivalent of being reassigned to a military base in the Arctic for being a troublesome child. That's about the best that will happen to you. The worst is it's easier for someone to step out of the shadows with a shotgun and turn you into hash rather than risk getting hurt confronting you head-on. Being violent at the drop of a hat may look really effective at the moment, but I've seen too many sheets with lumps under them in the middle of the street not to know what eventually comes of this attitude.

For grunts like us, "the pen and the sword in accord" works a whole lot better. Diplomacy without the force to back it up is useless, while force without thought is a nightmare. Each has its strengths and limitations. When used together, they complement each other and cover each other's weaknesses.

When you use diplomacy, there has to be an incentive for the other party to remain reasonable and compromise. If not, it's easier for the other guy to just use violence to get what he wants. The incentive is if you can't find a solution that is beneficial to both (important qualifier that, folks), you're going to hit him so hard that his momma's gonna fall down. If he knows that by becoming unreasonable he will end up in a world of hurt, that's a big incentive not to go there. There is even more incentive for him to behave if you let him know there is a chance he can get what he wants if he negotiates. But, unless he knows that he can't get away with being unreasonable, he WILL go off on you.

This is why having both the pen and the sword is a major factor in getting the number of conflicts that don't go physical to that 90-percent ratio.[5]

The tricky part is knowing when it's time to put down the pen and pick up the sword. That is to say, recognizing when it's gone to the 10 percent. When it's time to talk, you shouldn't be swinging fists and throwing kicks. When the time to talk is over, it's time for action. You do what you have to do, no hesitation, no regret. Learning the right time for each is a homework assignment that makes up a large part of your grade.

I'll give you a hint, though. The times for violence are few and far between. They seldom if ever involve strong emotion on your part. If you're feeling extremely angry or upset, odds are that isn't the right time. It's probably better to back off and get some distance from the situation until you cool down.

When someone commits physical violence against you, it is NOT the time for half-measures or debate. Most people are victimized by attackers because they're still thinking about being reasonable and negotiating while the guy is attacking. Once a situation turns physical, the time for talk is over. It has been taken to the next level. Drop diplomacy like an annoyed tarantula and shift to physical. I once heard about a test missile that had to be blown up in mid-flight because the engineers discovered, to their horror, that someone had failed to put an "end task" command in one of its programs. Once the program was launched, they couldn't stop it. Without that stop command, you had a wild and uncontrollable missile just whipping right along. That's why they had to blow it out of the sky. Because of this little glitch, with a push of a button, millions of dollars in equipment underwent instant disassembly. When to stop is just as important as when to go.

Let's address the issue of reasonable force. Most people tend to go overboard when it comes to defending themselves, and it gets them in trouble because they don't know when to stop! What constitutes "reasonable force" tends to vary from state to state, and I highly recommend you talk to a lawyer before you ever consider using your martial arts. If not, then at least go to the library and look up the specifics of your state's self-defense laws.

While it's not legal advice, here's a pretty good standard on what is reasonable use of force. You have the right to do whatever you need to do to stop an attacker. But once he's down, you can't jump up and down on his chest in a pair of spike heels." (OK, so it's from a women's self-defense course, but you have to admit the idea of some of those martial arts movie studs in high heels is kind of funny.)

That is a good rule of thumb. As long as the guy is attacking, you are "in the right" doing what is necessary to halt the attack. But once he goes down, you are legally required to stop. He is no longer an immediate threat.[6]

Another time people seriously blow it is when the guy turns away. Yes, he instigated an attack. But after you play "Rock 'em Sock 'em" Robots on his head a few times, he may decide that it wasn't such a bright idea after all. Hightailing it out of there suddenly begins to look real appealing, and he'll turn to do just that. At that moment, he is no longer attacking you, which means you are legally required to stop! If you don't, you are now attacking him. This is where that predator/blitzkrieg/werewolf training can and WILL get you in trouble. You gotta know when to stop. Whether the guy curls up to keep from getting hurt or is turning to run away, his attack is done.

It's obvious that whoever wrote these laws didn't have much first-hand fighting experience. Nor will the person prosecuting you have compassionate understanding. Believe me, it's incredibly easy to go over this fine line when you're scared, pumped up on adrenaline, and mixed up in the middle of a fight. Your amygdala[7] is running full steam ahead and, as far as it's concerned, the fact that the guy is still there means he's still attacking. It doesn't matter which way he's facing. Not true, but ye olde monkey brain thinks so.

This is why you need to add in an important command to your fight program. That is: RUN! Only engage in physical violence long enough to punch a hole to escape through.

I'm not talking Little Bunny Fufu running— where you dash around the edge of the room trying to avoid the big bad man. That will get you hurt. What I'm talking about has a serious edge to it, as in meet Fluffy the Cat. Have you ever tried to hold on to Fluffy in a vet's office when a large dog walked in? It's kind of amazing how such a small animal can create a sudden and serious need for oh-so-many stitches. That's because Fluffy's version of running isn't the same as Little Bunny Fufu's. Fluffy's attitude is that he will use your face as traction to get the hell out of there. What is scary is that his taking your eye out in the process is a side issue!

That's the kind of running I'm talking about. If you've ever been torn up in this manner, you already know that when you're holding onto something that is dedicated to getting out of there, it doesn't matter that you're 15 times its body weight. You get hurt and get hurt bad. Now, imagine how much damage something close to your own body weight could cause if it were equally dedicated to climbing over you. That's what you're going to do to your attacker. Ask any cop, hospital orderly, or mental health worker what is harder to handle: someone attacking you or someone dedicated to climbing over you to escape. Those of us who have been there know the damage this can cause.

When faced with such a situation, winning is no longer the issue for your attacker. He's going to be more concerned about not getting torn up. It's not something he can block because anything he puts out there to block with gets used as traction. He's got two hands, but you have two hands and two feet that are all being used to scramble over him. He sticks an arm out there, and you grab onto it and pull yourself over it. All of a sudden, he's down to one limb to fend off your three. Are you beginning to see why the Fluffy approach is such a mutha' to deal with? He's going to get seriously hurt as a by-product!

This "Get out of Dodge" mentality is especially needed when you're facing more than one opponent. The second you get past the guy in front of you, you go for breaking the land speed record. Until that time, it's no-holds-barred, tooth, nail, and fang to claw your way out. You're fighting for your safety, and that doesn't entail hanging around any longer for more things to go wrong.

Even if they follow you, it's going to be hard for them to convince the judge that they chased you in self-defense. Realistically though, most times they won't really chase you. They may give it a short go, but they often give up after a bit. Chasing someone who just used their friend's face for traction really isn't an appealing option. It's like chasing a tiger bare-handed. Do you really want to catch him?[8]

One of the main differences between you and a professional thug is that he has no hesitation about using violence. He can just walk away from the damage he causes. It's no sweat to him. He gets what he wants and leaves. He's not going to stay around and say, "Yes, that's the person I shot." Odds are, it's going to be a little harder for you to do the same. Many people are attacked near their homes, cars, work, or places where they regularly socialize. Witnesses will say, "I don't know the guy on the ground, but Joey Fettucini lives upstairs on the third floor." Oops.

Chances are good that you will have to deal with the repercussions of physical violence. Unless you are so far into a lifestyle where violence is both common and not reported because everybody is involved in something they shouldn't be, you will end up talking to the cops. As I said before, the dirt-bag will lie. He has nothing to lose, but you do.

A bully will move on you without fear of repercussion if you are a stranger to the area. A person in an emotional state (or intoxicated) isn't thinking about the ramifications of his actions, either. The only things he is reacting to are his immediate emotion and his desire to win, not the long-term consequences of his actions. In both cases, you're dealing with someone who doesn't care how much damage he does. But how much damage you do can get you into lots of trouble.

Physical damage, emotional damage, legal ramifications, and revenge-seekers all contribute to the aftermath of violence. Plan for these kinds of complications when you think about self-defense situations. You not only have to survive the assault, but what comes after it. This is a reality of self-defense that is seldom addressed by martial arts instructors: You might just have to defend yourself in court, so you'd better have your ducks in a row beforehand.

These days I teach a violence de-escalation program called "Assaultive Behavior Management." I'm going to pull a few points from it to help you understand what you're dealing with when you're confronting a violent person. If you really think you can afford to risk getting your face pushed in because you're such a whiz on how humans behave, go ahead and skip to the next chapter. If you feel, like I do, that it's better to swallow pride than blood, read on.

A number of years ago, I was having a conversation with one of the smartest men I have ever had the pleasure to know. He was a fascinating character who put himself through medical school by hiring out as a mercenary down in Central America. So you might say he was knowledgeable about the subject of conflict. We were talking shop, and he asked me, "If I were to hit you what would I be doing?"

"Other than signing your death warrant?" I asked flatly. (There are certain situations I don't like. Not even hypothetically.) When he answered in the affirmative, I sat there and thought about it for a few more moments. "You'd be telling me that you're pissed."

"Exactly," he responded. "I'd be communicating with you."

What occurred afterward was a long meandering conversation about the nature of communications that almost melted my brain. But the more I thought about it, the more sense that comment about communicating made.

What is important to realize is violence is a form of communication. It's just not with words. Many people are not familiar with this type of communication. When they encounter it, they go, "homina, homina, homina!" Way too many times, I've seen people reeling back in confusion from blows that weren't that hard instead of blocking the next attack. Being punched in anger is a serious shock, and they "shut down" while trying to figure out how to handle it. In the meantime, the Great Orator is all over them like white on rice. Boom, boom, boom, conversation over.

Let's go back to the beginning of the chapter. The reason I could take that guy's punch is that I am well-versed in the lingo of physical confrontation. Getting hit is not an overwhelming event to me. Nor is getting hit by an angry person (and believe me, there is a difference). It's just a message that things have changed a level. While the physical impact may be a shock to my system, both the message and the medium are old hat. "Oh gee, he's angry . . . oh me, oh my (yawn)." I know how to internally deal with such a message, and I'm not overwhelmed by shock when it happens. This also means that I'm not going to stand there and let him get in more of the same message. "Yeah, yeah, I heard you the first time, putz."

This is why it is important to get over your fear of getting hit. When they hear me say this, many people think I'm talking about going out and training in a hard-core, head-thumping, brain-bashing fashion all the time. Au contraire, mon ami. You don't have to do it all the time (that's liable to get you hurt more than anything else). What it does mean is that, for a while, you need to learn what it feels like to get punched hard and keep on going. You can take a punch and not be overwhelmed.

Now that's only one part of the message. I'm also talking about getting hit with the emotional message that the guy is pissed. Your monkey brain is reacting to the emotional threat as well. In fact, it's going to be reacting to that more than it is to getting hit. Remember that black belt who sat down when attacked for real? That was what was happening.

I seriously suggest you read Appendix B before going any further for a rundown on how our monkey brain reacts to emotional threat. Unless you are in a situation where you deal with aggressive behavior on a regular basis, you're going to have this emotional reaction. That is why scenario-based training is so good—it trains you both physically and emotionally.

If you can't afford to go through a course, talk with your sensei or training partner and do some training where they act angry and pop you with some force. Once you and your amygdala learn that you can take a serious emotionally charged punch and keep on going, it loses some of its fright value. Sure it hurts, but you can take it and still function. That's what you need to know. Learn to speak the lingo, and all of a sudden it becomes a whole lot less scary.

Let me stress that once you know that you can

take such a blow, turn the volume back down to prevent injuries.

As I said before, violence is a method of communication. It most often means that the guy is done being reasonable and is resorting to physical means to get his way. That "get his way" part defines one of the greatest motivations: Violence is a form of behavior for someone trying to get what he wants.

While there can be fruitcake violence—like the guy in the loony bin who suddenly freaks out thinking that little green lizards are coming out of the wall—99 percent of violence is based on the person using it to achieve a certain goal. What that goal is varies drastically from person to person, but this fact remains consistent. This even applies to the guy in the rubber room—he thinks by being violent he can prevent those nasty lizards from getting him.

Generally, most "fights" are about getting another person to conform to your standards and expectations of behavior. Whether the goal is an external one (i.e., "I will get you to behave by being violent") or an internal one (i.e., "I'll hurt you physically as punishment for hurting me emotionally") is totally dependent on the circumstances and the people involved.

The most common form of violence is one person enforcing his standards of behavior on another. Someone slugging someone else out of fury is an example of an assailant punishing unacceptable behavior. Whether that punishment is to keep the person from ever doing it again or just to make the slugger feel better is immaterial. The guy is engaging in violent behavior to get what he wants.

Knowing this goal gives you one of the best tools for preventing it. Simply let the person know that the violent behavior won't give him the results he wants. Not only won't he reach his goal, but he'll end up farther away than if he tried another means. I'm not talking about responding with a counterthreat of, "Oh yeah? I'll kick your butt!" I'm talking responding to someone's threat of violence by letting him know "You can't get there from here." It's not a matter of winning or losing, it's simply that you will not get the results you want from this course of action.

Want to know the absolute worst type of fighter to go up against? It's not the guy who's determined to win at all costs. It's the one who's determined that if he doesn't win, neither will you. He may go down, but he'll take you with him.

Let me tell you from personal experience that developing this demeanor will do wonders for keeping you out of fights. Not only is it one of the best ways of making sure that the person doesn't get what he wants by being violent, but it lets him know, win, lose, or draw, that it's going to cost him. While they may not know the term, the idea of a Pyrrhic victory—a victory won at overwhelming expense—is well known among those who use violence. And they don't want to mess with it.

Many people who use violence come at it from the standpoint of the more they crank up the volume, the better the chances they have of getting what they want. They win, they walk away with all the marbles, and that is that. This is why the game escalates. Both parties pump up the volume. If you threaten them with you winning, then you are playing the same game. This is the classic, "I'm going to kick your butt!" "Oh yeah, I'll kick yours!" From that standpoint, it's just a matter of who can crank up the volume fast enough to win. It assumes that whoever wins is going to get his way. There is no incentive not to escalate the situation to violence.

On the other hand, what happens when someone calmly says, "Yeah, you can kick my butt, but I'll take you down with me"? All of a sudden what that guy is expecting to get out of winning is no longer there. Even if he wins, he's going to be seriously hurt. Win, lose, or draw, he's going to get hurt. What benefit he was hoping to get out of becoming violent isn't there anymore.

The samurai made a big production about going out to battle and being ready to die. Well, I'm Scottish, and we make a bigger deal out of revenge. Like badgers, we believe that anyone who sticks a hand into our burrow needs to be informed about the error of his ways by pulling back a bloody stump. The idea isn't that I'm ready, willing, and able to die (any idiot can do that), but that no matter what happens I'm going to make the guy pay a high price for behaving in this way. You may kill us, but it's going to cost you big time.

Believe it or not, this is better for keeping you out of trouble than being willing to die. See, someone who isn't afraid to die is easily obliged by just shooting him. You can shoot someone who is bent on avenging himself on you all you want, but that still isn't going to keep him from burying his teeth in your throat and taking you with him. With this in mind, how likely are you to pick a fight with such a person? Well, neither are the bad guys.

ANIMAL'S IMPORTANT SAFETY TIP

- People who use violence have to accept the fact that violence can be returned onto them. Most, however, skate along in the firm belief that if they use violence first, they will win. Mostly this is true. The average person hesitates about using violence even to defend himself. It is a deeply ingrained civilized response. We were taught that it's wrong to use violence to win our way. Unfortunately, laughing boy has not only forgotten that, but he has discovered that he can get away with using violence.

Ed Parker once said in describing the outcome of a fight, "It's not who's right, but who's left." Unfortunately, history tends to agree with him, as who was right was often determined by who was left standing after the battle. The guy who is trying to pick a fight with you is only concerned with what he wants, not what you want, and he's willing to use violence to get it. The best way to keep him from trying anything violent on you is to let him know that he can't get away with it. No matter what. Even if he wins, he won't be around to enjoy the fruits of his victory.

While this sounds like I am contradicting what I said earlier about escape being your goal, I'm not. Plan A is to get out of there. It just so happens that what you're going to use as traction is his face. In escaping, you're going to cause damage. But if you can't escape, making him hurt is Plan B. Nine times out of 10 though, Plan A is going to cause so much damage to him, he's not going to be real interested in seeing your Plan B.

It doesn't matter how afraid you are, how mad you are, or how much you desperately don't want to be there. As long as you keep in mind the goal that if you are trapped, you will do everything in your power not to win but to hurt the other person as badly as he's hurting you, you will be able to deter most conflicts.

The reason all of this works as a deterrent is simple. It shows the other person that violence is the wrong choice of behavior to get what he wants. It's too high a price to pay. But once he stops, you stop, whether you're fighting with bare hands or weapons. You don't escalate the situation, you just stop it.

Let's Get the Rules Straight

45

Once you firmly entrench this goal in your head a whole mess of fear, confusion, and trepidation goes out the window. It also drastically affects how you communicate with the person offering you violence. This is because your body language changes. There is an indefinable but important change that comes over how you present yourself, how you stand, how you look, and how you sound when you have this goal firmly entrenched in your mind. Somehow, it conveys itself to the other person.

You communicate with him that you are no longer an easy victim. There's just something about you that tells him, "Better leave this one alone." Believe it or not, even if you're terrified there's something about you that will say, "This one is scared enough to hurt me badly." Kinda takes the fun out of scaring someone doesn't it?

As you progress and get more experience with successfully using this mind-set, you can change it from "no matter what happens I'll get a hunk out of you" to an even better one for stopping violence from occurring. That is, "It ain't gonna happen, Buckaroo." All sorts of things aren't going to work out the way laughing boy wants them to. He's not going to kick your butt. He's not going to get his way. He's not going to walk away unscathed. He's not going to win. He's not going to overwhelm you. Most importantly, violence isn't going to get him what he wants. And the harder he tries to force the issue, the harder he's going to hit the ground being told NO! And all of this isn't a threat—it's just the way it is.

Notice that neither of these mind-sets are focused on your "winning" through violence. They aren't about starting violence to get your way. What they are is focused on keeping him from starting violence to get his way. If he's going to win and get his way, it's through something other than the use of violence.

What I want to address now is being afraid. Personally, I consider this to be an excellent emotion and don't recommend you try to get rid of it, or worse, worry about how it makes you look to others. Fear can make you a better fighter. Yep, it's true. Don't think that being afraid is a bad thing. In fact, like that character in David Gemmell's novel said, it can be a good thing. If it's the right kind.

For years and years, I was embarrassed by the fact that I was afraid in many of the situations I found myself in. I mean, I was so scared that afterward I went out and threw up. Thing was, people kept on telling me how impressed they were that I was so fearless. (Yeah, right, you ought to see what it looks like from this side, folks). Truth was I was so scared that I was moving with blinding speed and incredible power. When I blocked with lightning speed, it wasn't because I was a kung fu master, *it was because I was afraid of getting hurt!* The reason I crawled all over the dude wasn't because I was a master of karate, it was because I didn't want him to hurt me! If I was hitting him that much, he wasn't about to be able to hit me, now was he? Ergo, I'd Taz out on the dude. It always surprised me how little I got hurt when my actions were powered by near blind panic.

Like I said before, it is really difficult to stop someone who is bound and determined to leave the scene by crawling over you. It's one thing to catch someone who's trying to scoot past you and quite another to stop someone who's climbing over you using tooth, claw, and toenails for extra traction. Often I was just trying to get past someone when I suddenly realized I had hurt him so badly that he was no longer attacking. Kewl . . .

So don't worry about being scared. It's the smart thing to do. But use your fear to achieve the end of getting out of there by crawling over his face. Let him know you are so scared of him that you will do something drastic to his precious body while getting away from him. Using your fear this way keeps you from falling into the "I'm a scared little bunny that is easy prey" mind-set that so many victims have. You might as well write "free lunch" on yourself and go skinny-dipping with a school of piranha, because that attitude is guaranteed to get you attacked. That is the kind of person who zips around like a fish in an aquarium trying to dodge the net instead of coming over it. Bullies, thugs, rapists, and criminals love to see this attitude, because they know they've got you on the run already.

Want to know something scary? I've seen this most with people who are trying to stand up for themselves. It's the person who's obviously thinking to himself, "I'm terrified but maybe if I stand up to them like a manly man they'll leave me alone" who plays right into the hands of the bad boys. They love this kind of person. When you're standing there with your knees knocking and every nerve in your body screaming "RUN!" how convincing do you think you're going to be about not being afraid of them? Believe me, they will call your bluff. Then what are you going to do? Worse, while you're standing there bravely, they're moving into perfect attack position. Get blindsided upside the head with a bottle and it doesn't matter if you're scared or not. Once again, they've got you.

On the other hand, the guy who is so scared that he's going to go off on the bad boy if he makes a threatening move is a whole different enchilada. He poses a danger, while the would-be tough guy trying to hide his fear doesn't.

Other people make the serious mistake of trying to avoid violence by trying outdo the guy threatening them. Instead of sitting back with an "it ain't gonna happen" attitude, they end up getting right back in the guy's face, hoping to chase him off. They end up actually causing a situation to explode rather than de-escalating it by hitting the guy with an attitude of "You're going to kick my butt? No way, dude! I'm going to kick yours!" In doing so, they become overly blusterous and aggressive, which in turn causes the guy to go off.[9]

While there are a few situations that can be resolved by jumping back in the guy's face, they are much rarer than you'd think. If you've been a good boy or girl, these kinds of situations are few and far between. You don't avoid violence by playing the same game as the other guy. All that does is convince him that he needs to crank up the volume in order to win. Usually this translates in his mind into, "In order for me to get what I want, I'd better hit him now." Not exactly the reaction you were hoping for was it?

This is why you need take your amygdala out for a cup of coffee. Sit down and explain to it that it has a new set of orders. The second the guy makes a move to attack you, it's to take every tool you have learned in the martial arts and every ounce of fear it has and jet out of there. It's OK to use laughing boy's face for traction, but leave the scene you will. Trust me, these are the kind of orders it can understand REAL well.

---

[1]   STBY: Sucks To Be You

[2]   After a few of those occasions, it becomes obvious that what you thought was a funny, witty comment is not universally thought so by your fellow man.

[3] I've also noticed that these people like to think they can say anything they want. When that is proven untrue, they run to mommy as well. They can use their weapons to hurt you, but they get upset if you respond, especially if you use different tools.

[4] See *Violence, Blunders and Fractured Jaws,* à la me.

[5] I could have said negotiate from a position of strength, but many people read that as, "I tell you what to do." To them, negotiation is just the guy dragging his feet before he accepts their will. That is not negotiation. It is, however, a great way to guarantee that the guy busts you one in the face. The person who negotiates that way doesn't let the other guy save face. The goal of negotiation is mutual benefit, even if it is as basic as "I let you live, you let me live." Which, when you're dealing with a mugger in a parking lot, is a real successful way to go.

[6] Well . . . maybe in an ideal world. Truth is, if you stand over him, he can attack again. On the other hand something as simple as backing away (oh wow, what a concept!) can nullify any potential threat while he's on the ground. The problem with this is people on the ground have a nasty habit of getting up—which puts you right back where you started from. But, if you split before he can get up . . . even better.

[7] Basically, your monkey brain. Turn to Appendix B right now for a very important rundown on how your brain ticks. There's a lot of information in it that should affect how you train.

[8] Of course what happens in the following weeks is another story. It just so happens I know this guy who wrote a book called *Street E & E: Evading, Escaping, and Other Ways to Save Your Ass When Things Get Ugly.* Hint, hint, nudge, nudge.

[9] As an important safety tip, this is especially common with women and rape. Many women get verbally violent in trying to get the guy away from them and actually end up infuriating the guy more. If you aren't willing to back it up physically, win, lose, or draw, don't verbally provoke someone, especially rapists, since the guy is already looking for an excuse to go off.

Oh, What a Difference a Day Made

....

You can tell he ain't never been in combat, he wants to fight.
—WWII cartoonist Bill Mauldin's "Willie & Joe" watching as a spit-and-polish soldier swaggers past

"How many knife fights have you been in?"
"I've studied kali for 15 years under master . . ."
"That's not what I asked. I asked how many actual knife fights have you been in?"
"Well, I'm trained in five styles of knife fighting . . ."
Sigh

Around this time in these conversations, I begin to have an overwhelming urge to put my head down and rub my eyes. Yeah, I'm dealing with a real knife fighter here. I know because his business card says so, right there. Having survived more than a few situations where someone tried to play show and tell with my internal organs, I can say that a majority of what this so-called knife-fighter is teaching is functionally useless in the real thing. It's entirely too sophisticated—and therefore subject to failure—for real-world application.

I want to point out something strange here. Having survived the real thing a few times, if I met Mr. Knife Fighter in an alley, I would be the one walking out of there. Inversely, however, in an academy or school that same kali guy would cream me in a point-based sparring match. Under "controlled conditions," I'd lose. We're talking a point spread as bad as if the Green Bay Packers took on a peewee football team. Victory, it seems, becomes almost purely situational. So where does this paradox come from?

Let me ask you a question about sparring. And in answering it, you'll know the answer to both questions. How many times have you tried a technique that just didn't work out the way you planned?

I'll bet dollars to doughnuts that you have some really neat sneaky move up your sleeve that you like to pull on opponents during sparring matches. Realistically, however, unless the circumstances are juuuuuuuust right, this smoking move only has a 1-in-3 chance of working. If it doesn't work, you step back and wait for another chance to use it later. Or you step back and let your opponent get all hairless about that weird move that came out of nowhere and almost got him. I've seen many people overprotect themselves against such a move happening again. In doing so, they leave other targets open. (This is why I say sparring strikes are for points or psychological damage.)

Sparring is fighting with Goldilocks fu. That means you want to use a move that isn't too hot or too cold, too hard or too soft. You have the time to find the one that's just right. It may take you a few times, but eventually you'll be awarded a point using that move. The problem is, in the real thing you only get one shot.

That's because laughing boy there is using Br'er

Bear fu. All he wants to do is bash you on the head. This changes the entire picture. Nine times out of 10, the outcome of a fight is determined by who hits first and causes the most damage fastest. While the two are often synonymous—as many a fast, light puncher has discovered while being picked up and thrown over the pool table—this is not always the case.

This is one reason why I walk out of alleys but can lose on the mat. I'm not a speed fighter. As long as you stretch it out, break it up, and there is no real damage being done, then the better technician *will* win. He will take the points. It looks like he's beating the hell out of me, but it's not truly effective.

Let me give you an analogy. Years ago, my brother and I used to go out topless-bar crawling on our motorcycles. I was on a 250 Yamaha while he had his Harley. As long as we were on the city streets where there were stoplights, I could beat him off the line every time. I'd be sitting at the next light grinning evilly at him and making comments that he needed to feed the poor, tired squirrel he had in the engine. As long as we had short scramble conditions where I could zip off the line then stop, I'd dust him again and again. However, when we'd get on the highway and he could unwind that mother, he'd leave me so far behind that he looked like a dot. By the time I got to where we were going, he'd be well into his first beer, relaxed, and enjoying the ladies. Then it was my turn to put up with comments about how even a tired, hungry squirrel is better than little itty-bitty mice.

I had the speed getting off the line, but my bike didn't have power. As long as there was a stoplight up ahead, I was real cocky. Take that stoplight away, though, and I didn't even have what it took to keep up, much less win. The sparring ring is like my little Yamaha. It's a series of races from stoplight to stoplight. There, speed without power wins. But in a real fight, where there aren't any stoplights, power becomes real important. All it takes is one twist of the throttle by Bubba and the issue is over.

You may be faster than greased lightning in the ring, but it's the guy who does the most damage quickest who's going to walk out of the alley. I'll tell you right now that few people are fast and powerful. They're usually one or the other, not both.[1]

The second major difference between street-fighting and martial arts is complexity. The secret to effective fighting in the street is K.I.S.S. (keep it simple, stupid). In the real thing, simple moves tend to be more effective because that's all you have time for! Remember what I mentioned before about a favorite technique that only works one out of three times? You don't want to use those sorts of things. What you want are simple, powerful, bulletproof moves that work when you have some ape trying to eat your face. Those fancy moves tend to crash on their own anyway. But how much more likely are they to glitch when the guy is not only attacking you, but actively trying to make your attempts to stop him from chewing off your nose fail?! Letting you block his attacks is not on his list of things to do today. All it takes to keep you from blocking is to grab your arm, pull it out of the way, and punch.

Trust me, this tends to complicate things.

Don't think these aren't critical factors in the real thing. In a nutshell, you're only going to have about three moves to prevent some knuckle-dragger from doing a polka on your face. You don't want to burn them up on ineffectual moves. You only got so much time, don't waste it.

Those are just some of the differences between sparring and the real thing. Another is intent. I don't care if it's bare handed, weapons, full contact, or point sparring—intent is a major difference. Perhaps the biggest of all. No matter how intense a sparring match can get, the guy you are facing isn't out to hurt you. He may be out to win. And he may even be looking to peg you a couple of good ones over and above what is necessary, but he is not intent on causing you serious bodily damage, whereas in a real fight, your opponent is trying to do just that. And that, mi amigo, is a BIG difference.

It's one thing to go at it full force within the restrictions and rules of a tournament. You do this knowing full well that there are judges there who will intervene if things get too wild. Under these circumstances, if things really get out of hand, maybe a bone will get broken. It's quite another to have the gut-wrenching realization that the howling, barking, drooling maniac coming at you means you serious injury. The least he wants to do is break something. One situation's extreme is the other's minimum.

That shock is made worse by another chilling realization: In the real thing, there's nothing between you and him except air. No judges, no rules, and nobody else there to stop him. It's the difference between seeing a lion safely behind bars at a zoo and having a hungry one suddenly charging out of the bushes at you. All of a sudden, it really is just you and him. If that doesn't scare the bejeebers out of you, you're not paying attention. You can train all you want, even to the point of being a real fire-eater in the dojang, but the first time you face someone with this intent, it will hit you like a 2x4 across the teeth. At that moment, it's no longer a matter of what you can do to him, but what he can do to you. That's when mortality comes knocking, and you realize "the real thing is not a game."

How you react to this intent is what spells the difference between coming out intact and getting seriously hurt. Some people actually freeze like a deer in headlights. Most, however, don't totally freeze. What they do is stand there and grope around trying to find what seems to be the best answer. Still, the end result of both is that the person doesn't do anything in time to stop an attacker. Both are disastrous reactions. This is part of what I was talking about when I said people defeat themselves in real fights.[2]

In general, people tend to react out of habit to the game they are familiar with. It's a human kind of thing to do. When the abnormal shows up they usually end up going, "homina, homina, homina," or they try to take it back to the more familiar. If you've ever seen people in a crisis situation, you'll know what I'm talking about. Many so-called gawkers are, in fact, frozen in shock. Some of the weirdest behavior you'll see in utter chaos is someone trying to put the world back to normal in a small but familiar way.[3] More specifically, while martial artists may be accustomed to punches coming at them, it's usually under very controlled circumstances. Seldom do these punches come at them in odd places and with intent. Under these circumstances, they either freeze or want to stand back and spar. This would take it back to "normal." Unfortunately, this leaves you wide open to getting the snot beaten out of you.

Until now we've been talking about how his intent affects you. But there is another side to the story and that is how it affects him. When someone goes postal on you, odds are he's willing to pay the price of your getting a few shots in on him before he overwhelms you. Usually, what he's banking on is that you'll hit like a girl. His plan is to get in fast and hard and start tap dancing on your face before you can crank up the volume and do it to him. Add to that, he's got an adrenaline rush that's going to mute out minor pain messages until he finishes stomping you. The problem is, by deciding to move first, he's got the jump on you with that adrenaline rush. It's pumping inside of him already. In other words, if you don't hit him with something hard enough to override his internal message of "kill him" (i.e., you), he's going to keep on coming. There are only a few seconds to do so before he lands on your face.

If you follow your sparring training and pull your punch, punch and pause, avoid hitting vital targets, or just stand back and spar, your blows won't stop the guy. You're burning your few moves with things that won't keep him off you. What would score you a solid point in the ring will just bounce off a committed attacker, and he'll keep on coming. Don't worry, though, once he's standing on your face, he'll probably content himself with just doing the Berkeley Stomp.[4]

Understand, if his intent is to hurt you, he wants to do it NOW! He especially doesn't want to fight you. He doesn't want to string it out, swap a few punches, take his time or make it last. No. He wants to do it this instant. His fist, your face. No waiting, no interference, and no delays. To achieve this, he'll be on you like white on rice. He's looking for a hole to bulldoze through so he can start whomping on you. If you leave one open, he'll come blasting through like a buffalo with an attitude to get to you. Guess what? Not having defenses that can handle a full-out charge constitutes having a major hole. Once this happens, you'll be on the retreat with little to no chance of recovering. This kind of fighting is not real subtle, but it is REALLY effective. And it is what most real fights are like.

Using tournament and sparring techniques in a real fight is like trying to fix your car with plumbing tools. They aren't useless tools. In fact, they are great tools for their specific environment—but they aren't designed to fix a carburetor. In short, you need the right tools for the task at hand. *You need to know when to use which set of tools!* Keeping the different groups of tools separate in your head is a *whole* lot more complicated than people think it is, especially for someone who has never been in a real fight, which most martial artists haven't been.

It's easy to think that all you do is turn up the volume on a blow, but the truth is you have years of training using other tools. It's a totally different set of physics, a different mind-set, and a different set of motor skills to be able to hit an angry, charging person in a vital area hard enough to stop him.

Welcome to the jungle, kids. Unlike Elias from *Platoon*, though, I'm going to tell you why I'm pulling things off you. By the end of this book, you will understand the differences between street and dojo. Then you will be able to tailor your martial arts training to fit your needs and the needs of your students to stay alive in the real thing. Even if you don't agree with what I say, you will have a better understanding of the issues that contribute to the problem of making martial arts work on the street.

---

[1] Momentum = Mass x Velocity. Plucking a number out of the air, let's say momentum is 12. Basically, you can get there in one of two ways. Make mass either 3 or 4 and make velocity the corresponding number. That's an OK hit. However, what most people do is 6 x 2. They put everything into either mass (power) or velocity (speed). When they crank it up, what they get is 12 x 1. That's lacking in critical elements, whereas a more balanced (and effective) hit can be easily cranked up to 6 x 6. That's both fast and damaging. Remember, it's not just

speed or power, but who does the most damage the fastest that counts. I'll go more into how to achieve this later.

[2] See Appendix B to learn about the physical mechanism of your brain and why stress training is so important.

[3] In the movie *Gone with the Wind*, with the Union Army shelling Atlanta just hours away from invading, a woman is having complications birthing a baby, and everything is just generally going to hell in a hand basket. Aunt Pitty-Pat, a fat old society woman, is running around in circles ranting that what Scarlett is doing isn't "proper ladylike behavior." That's an example of trying to bring an out-of-control situation back to "normal" by fixating on something small and insignificant.

[4] That's where you put the open mouth of a downed opponent around a curb and kick the back of his head.

CHAPTER 4

What You're Up Against

....

Your first goal isn't to win;
your first goal is not to lose

—Lil' ol' me

In the movie *Dazed and Confused,*[1] there is really good representation of what most fights really are vs. what most people think they will be. A kid who is not a fighter, but who lost face when he backed down from a tough guy, decides he must do something to avenge his honor. After a long bout of talking himself into it, he walks up to the tough dude and just decks him with a sucker punch.

However, instead of completing the process by doing a fandango on the guy's face, he just stands there in a macho fighting stance. The tough guy gets up and throws himself on the kid with a flurry of punches. He rides the hapless kid down to the ground and proceeds to knock the snot out of him until other partygoers pull him off.

Welcome to reality, kid. Most real fights are sudden, fast, and brutal. They are not really complicated or sophisticated, nor are they displays of skill. One person (usually the attacker) blows a hole open in the other guy's defenses and proceeds to drive in as fast and hard as he can. For those of you who missed the reference, it means he's throwing multiple punches that are connecting, most often through the same hole he just created. Usually the other guy, unaccustomed to someone having a knees up on his face as he tries to walk backward, falls over. The first one continues to rain blows until he's satisfied or someone pulls him off his victim.

Not a whole lot of room for style and finesse there, but it is oh-so-effective. And odds are that's what you're going to be up against. How would your style hold up against this kind of attack? What if there were tables, chairs, other people, walls, or cars in the way? In case you haven't noticed, these things make walking forward interesting enough. They make trying to walk backward real difficult.

Herein lies the major problem, and it is the very problem that the kids in *Platoon* were facing. What you were trained for isn't necessarily what you're going to encounter out there. Actually, a more accurate way of saying it would be that what you've been trained to handle is only part of the problem, not the whole burrito. A real fight is when you see the rest of the Gut O' Hell Grande.

Over and above that particular problem, we have another. I'm always amazed with the selectivity of people who think stuff transfers over from the sparring ring to real fights. While a lot of stuff does translate over, unfortunately it's usually the stuff you don't want. How many times have you had things just go sideways in a sparring match? I mean nothing works right. Well, that's one of the things that *does* transfer over, and it does so with amazing efficiency.

Things do go wrong in the middle of a fight, and in a major way. Understand a big part of why Mr. Murphy[2] shows up is that the other guy is NOT cooperating with you! In fact, he's doing everything in his power to make things go another way! Under these circumstances, it's no wonder that things go wildly wrong—not only with complicated techniques, but even basic stuff. Unfortunately, while you're trying to figure out why it didn't work the way it did in the dojo, he's line dancing on your chest.[3]

Before you do unto him make sure he can't do unto you! Sound so obvious that it's idiotic? Well, I've seen many a bloody mess that used to be some stud who went into a fight thinking that he didn't have to worry because he was sure he was going to kick the other guy's butt right off.

ANIMAL'S IMPORTANT SAFETY TIP

- This has saved my life many times over. Consider what I am about to say very carefully because it's of vital importance. Its simplicity belies its profoundness. *You don't win a fight by being stronger than your opponent, you win by having fewer weaknesses.*

Sound like the same thing? It isn't. Think about it this way: Winning a fight isn't about how much damage you do to your opponent, but how much damage you keep him from inflicting on you. It's not just you getting through his defenses, but keeping him from getting through yours. Remember, it's not a one-way street; as you're flying at him, he's flying at you. That makes how well you attend to the weaknesses in your defenses pretty damned important. It's those weaknesses that he will come through to cause damage. Take my word for it on this one, this can really mess up your plans for victory. Sometimes this will happen just because he's a gorilla whose only intention is to crack your head wide open. Unknowingly, this ape has found a serious weakness in your defenses. Because often, you have unwittingly trained away from dealing with raw power attacks!

This is a common problem, and I have seen many people get their faces split open because of it. Think about it. How often do you throw just flat-out power attacks? The higher you advance, the more skill, control, and refinement go into your attacks. (It's called being good at your art, duhhh!) And the attacks you're used to dealing with from other advanced practitioners are also more and more refined. It can become a duel of subtlety, speed, and skill—like two guys with rapiers. It's motherin' fast and hard to follow with the naked eye.

It's not until you step in the ring with a white belt and get pegged a good one that you remember that there are people out there who use power instead of skill. While many try to pass it off as a "lucky shot," the fact that you're off in a corner, hunched over and trying to breathe through the pain should remind you how effective this type of attack can be. You just got your chimes rung by a white belt who wasn't out to hurt you. Want to guess what such an attack would be like if the guy throwing it *did* intend to hurt you? All of a sudden, that rapier meets up with a broadsword. CHOP!

That's just one example of the problems you're facing by switching from the dojang to the street. There are many, many more out there. The best way to Murphy-proof your defenses is to know the inherent strengths and weaknesses of your style. The number one thing to do is take a long, hard look at the emphasis your style puts on not getting hit. Trust me, this is a biggie. Styles that overemphasize what you're going to do to him tend to be real weak here. Granted, sometimes the best defense is a good offense, but experience has taught me that way too often laughing boy has the same philosophy, and they tend to clash. It's during that clash that the hole becomes apparent.

Let me go once again to the movies to illustrate a point. In *A Connecticut Yankee in King Arthur's Court*, Bing Crosby is supposed to joust. As he's standing there waiting, an armoured[4] guy with a lance sticking out of his chest is carried by on a stretcher. Crosby looks at the poor sod sympathetically and says, "Tough luck there, old boy." His buddy leans over and tells Bing, "That's the winner."

Oops. Big change of plans here, we're not going to play that game. Crosby then goes out and wins the joust. But he doesn't do it by suiting up in heavy armour and crashing head-on into his opponent. Instead, without armour, he gets on his faster, lighter pony and runs circles around the knight. He lets the tin man chase him around a bit and then ropes the knight off his horse. Big guy, big horse, heavy armour . . . fall down and go BOOM! Real hard. End of fight.

This is an example of weakness in one's strength—also known as a hole. For all of the knight's strength in armour, weight, protection, and ability to take a blow, where he was weak was in mobility, flexibility, and speed. While Crosby was nowhere near as strong as the knight, he didn't have the same weaknesses either. As long as he didn't go head-to-head with the battleship, he could win using a different approach. Bing won not by contesting his opponent's strength, but by exploiting his weaknesses. And it was a weakness created by the knight's very strength!

Now while we all want to be like Crosby, unfortunately most of us are like the knight. He was operating in a closed system. That means he was battling only with people who did things the same way he did. They'd get dressed up in boilerplate underwear and proceed to try to beat each other into unconsciousness. It was a strength-to-strength contest under strictly limited conditions. Under those conditions, this knight was a holy terror. But when he met up with someone who did things differently, he ended up sucking earth.

Notice the similarities between that sort of tournament and a martial arts tournament. Many styles are closed systems. Most of the sparring they do is intraschool or in tournaments against schools teaching the same style. Even if it's not the same style, the tourney rules tend to homogenize everything. It's not until something that is ordinarily verboten comes into play that you see exactly how limited the conditions of the tourney really are. If you take a look at the first few Ultimate Fighting Championships, that's exactly what happened. Everyone went in there expecting it to be a stand-up fight, and they got creamed when it went to the ground.[5] In your school, you get accustomed to fighting under certain circumstances—circumstances that will not be repeated out in the street. You can easily find yourself trying to chase a little guy on a pony.

The problem is that in the wild world of real violence, weakness in strength is really a rock/paper/scissors kind of thing. The strength of your style is like the rock—sometimes it will win; sometimes it will lose. It all depends on what you're up against.

Here's a little game you can play to illustrate this

point. Take from a deck of cards the aces and the kings, keeping them in two piles. Each suit will represent a different way of fighting. First take the ace of spades. That's the style you're trained in. While the ace is the highest card, it is only so in the case of the same suit. Shuffle up the two piles separately. Flip a card over from the king pile. If it is the king of spades, you've lucked out: The guy fights like you do. Your ace beats his king, and you win. If it's anything else, you've just gotten your butt kicked.

You can cross-train, which means you get to pull another ace out of the pile. Now you have two. Reshuffle the king pile, and this time pull out two cards. If you match both, you win. If only one matches, you have a 50-50 chance of winning. Toss a coin to see if you win or lose. Now toss the remaining aces into the king pile and shuffle. If you pull an ace, you lose. Before you continue to read, go out and try this game.

I'm going to assume that you've just come back from a rather unpleasant experience here. If you think the odds were unfair, let me remind you that there are four focuses in the martial arts. In addition there are the three ranges of fighting and weapons, and that again makes four. The odds of meeting someone who fights like you do are pretty much like that game. Slim to none and Slim left town.

By playing this game a few times, you'll quickly realize that the only way to win consistently is to cross-train in all sorts of different styles. And that means styles that have totally different emphases. It doesn't do you any good to know six styles that are basically the same. Great, now you have six aces of spades instead of one. It still doesn't help you against a king from another suit. You need aces in all suits. Let's call spades distance fighting, diamonds grappling, clubs weapons, and hearts infighting. That's what cross-training does. Each style addresses different issues of what you're likely to encounter out in the real thing.

Finding where your style does—and doesn't—work is the cornerstone to making your martial arts style street effective. Then you can take stuff from other systems that are strong in the areas where your style is weak and incorporate them into your own. The thing is, you're not going to learn your system's weaknesses from inside your own system! There are two ways to learn where your style is weak. One is by going to different dojos/dojangs/kwoons and seminars and cross-training (or work out with people from other styles). The other is to run into someone in an alley. The first is a much more pleasant way to learn.

Most real fights contain elements of the following: at least one extremely emotional and/or drunken participant, sudden blitzkrieg multiple attacks, and lousy lighting. Plus, they are either happening in cramped spaces or with major obstacles underfoot. There is also a tendency of having one or more participant ending up on the floor—usually because the combatants run into each other and fall over rather than as a result of hooks, throws, or secret fighting techniques. Under those conditions, you will either land on various items like chairs, tables, or bottles, or his friends will proceed to have a great time hootin,' hollerin,' and kicking your ribs in. This is what real fights are like.

With criminal violence, you might want to add "unexpected" and "with a weapon" to the list. The guy is asking for directions one minute and has a weapon in your face the next. Add to this that he also has no hesitation about pulling the trigger of the gun he's pointing at you. That seriously limits the time you have for any effective response. The

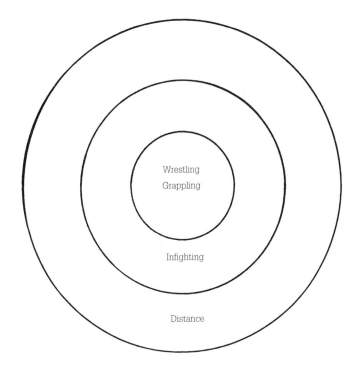

Circles of Distance

good news is that unless he's a rapist, he probably doesn't want to grapple.

If these descriptions don't rain on your parade in one way or the other, you must be an 87-year-old grandmaster. I'll tell you this, it's enough even to torque my wa (which it has. . . on many occasions). This is the difference between what you've trained for and reality.

The bottom line here, folks, is that no one style covers all of those variables![6] Look at those conditions. They're nasty! This is why you not only have to cross-train, but fieldstrip what you know to make it more workable under a wide array of circum-

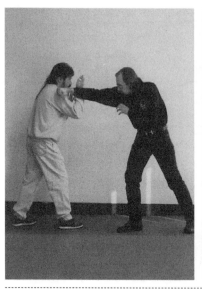
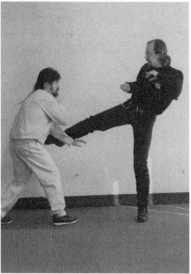

Distance punch   Distance kick

stances. Don't just learn different styles of the same thing, learn different styles that focus on different ranges, different philosophies, and different emphases.

Sticking with my old model, there are three ranges of fighting.[7]

- Distance
- Infighting
- Wrestling (now called "grappling"—remember, I wrote these books back in the pterodactyl days)

DISTANCE

Now, some folks use a four-range model, and I've even heard of five. But being an old belly scratcher, I prefer to stick to the easier-to-remember model of three. The ranges are simple—distance is between 2 and 5 feet away. It comprises long punches and

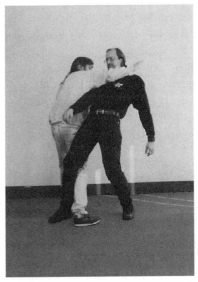
Grappling/wrestling

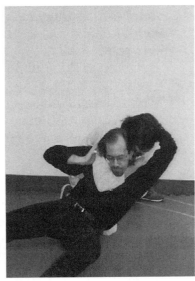
Grappling/judo

kicks (this is where some folks split the two types
of attacks and call them different ranges). You'll
probably recognize this as sparring range. This is
where people stand back and poke at each other.
Nothing wrong with that; it's a good sport range.
Most martial arts focus largely on this range.

GRAPPLING

Grappling you know about already. Whether you're
still on your feet while throwing someone or hitting
the deck with the guy, it's up close and personal.

It's also one of the most dangerous ranges to be
in during a street fight. Not because the guy could
Gracie Jujutsu you, but because a) his buddy could
pick up a chair and swat you like a bug, b) you
could crack your head open on the concrete when
you fall, c) you could land on a table or curb and the
combination of your weight and his could break

What You're Up Against 71

your back or drive a rib into your lungs, or d) his buddies could decide the night's entertainment is to kick you to death.

Going to the ground in a real fight is inviting a trip to the hospital. As there is a major difference between a real knife fight and playing in the dojo, there's a big difference between grappling in a tourney and doing it in a real confrontation in the street.[8]

INFIGHTING

Infighting is a much misunderstood distance. Most people think it's a small town you drive through on your trip to Grappling, Wisconsin. That is until they find someone who knows how to use it, such as a boxer, a wing chun practitioner, or a silat/kuntao fighter—then OUCH! Their car suffers a breakdown and they discover themselves at the mercy of a small-town mechanic.

Infighting occurs within a distance of anywhere between 6 inches and 2 feet. Unlike grappling, there is not usually body-to-body contact. Fist to body, elbow to body, forearm to body, knee to body, head-butting, yes; body to body, no. One of the secrets of keeping people in this range (instead of their crashing into you and grappling) is using your forearms as a buffer/shield. (In fact,

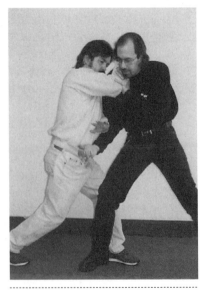

Infighting

imagining that you are using a shield is a good way to understand how to keep people off you.)

Perhaps the best thing that could be said about this range is it's a real fur ball. I mean it is nasty. But how well you handle this range is also where most fights (and tournaments) will be determined. It is here that you will either mess up a distance fighter or stop a grappler from getting his hands on you. Most importantly, however, it is here that you will stop an untrained bubba from closing with you and doing what that tough guy did to the kid in *Dazed and Confused.*

You must acquaint yourself with these three basic ranges and be somewhat capable in each. Look again at the idea of cross-training in different styles because each style addresses each range differently. Some styles are really strong in one range and pathetic in others. Other styles address the same range, but under entirely different conditions. Some are weapons-based and others are empty-hand.

Here's a set of gross generalizations about grappling arts that will get many practitioners really flamed, but it's worth looking at to understand the differences within a range: Aikido is great for avoiding attacks and taking wily hard-style fighters down. Even though it's technically grappling, most of it is done on your feet and at arm's length. Much of the judo I've seen is designed to work against the clinch that invariably happens during fights. It's knowing how to get the guy off you. It's done hip to hip, face to face. Like I said, it's for when the guy slams into you in the middle of a fight. The Brazilian Jujutsu practitioner often goes into a fight with the intention of taking it to the ground and fighting the guy into submission there. They intentionally slam into you to get you down where they can slap a joint lock or submission hold on.

Now, I will be the first to admit that is a horrible generalization, and there is much overlap among the arts and techniques. But you begin to see that even within a range there are drastic differences among styles. Now imagine how big a difference there is between styles that focus on different ranges! This is where cross-training really begins to make sense.

EXPECT THE UNEXPECTED

Another common scenario of a real fight is multiple attackers, often with one or more of them circling and attacking from behind. Street punks seldom operate alone, so you might as well assume that you're going to be facing more than one person in the real thing. If you train for that and you find yourself facing only one, it's a walk in the park.

Oh yeah, just to make it even more warm and fuzzy, add in a weapon to any of these scenarios. Edged weapons just have to touch you once in order to be effective. Even a fast, light strike can be devastating. Does your style teach you how to avoid being touched? Or does it tend toward having you take a punch to give one? How about my favorite fantasy move—do you train for disarming a person with a weapon? (*Snort* good luck.)

Or do you work on the more realistic approach of taking him out as he's drawing a concealed gun? Like Mike Haynack said, "I don't have to be faster than a bullet, I just have to be faster than the guy with the gun." That is a good thing to keep in mind, especially about your attack being faster than his draw.

POSITIVE THINKING

OK, let's look at this in a more positive light. You know the bad news already, so lets start putting figures in the good news column. Courtesy of Peyton Quinn's keen abilities in observation,[9] you get to know a really simple point that can do wonders for keeping you from getting your face pushed in. The two most common attacks you'll be facing are the straight punch and the hook. That's what is going to be coming at you the most in a real fight.

Let me add that most blows by untrained fighters will be to your face.[10] Even someone with lots of fighting experience will tend to follow this pattern. It's only after training (or lots and lots of experience) that people begin to focus the majority of their attacks elsewhere or use other blows.

Now what does this tell us? Well, aside from the fact that most people aren't real imaginative, it pretty much indicates where he's going to be pouring all of his energy. Consequently, a great deal of what we do should be devoted to keeping him from successfully breaking through our defenses when he is coming at us up high!

Chris Caracci[11] has a saying, "Train as you live, live as you train," which I agree with 100 percent. Like I've said, you will react according to your training. Chris's comment reflects the importance of correct training and consistency with reality. I have a saying along the same lines that is more focused on keeping my face from getting smooshed: "If you train for what happens most, you'll be able to handle most of what happens."

What is normally coming at you in a real fight isn't sophisticated, trained, or devious. It's more like a series of waves that will overwhelm and blow through your defenses. If you don't manage to handle the first wave, the rest are just going to keep on coming in and pounding you. You have to stop those waves—not only the first, but those coming immediately afterward.

What You're Up Against

Realize that once you figure out a way to keep from being immediately overwhelmed by its power, a wave is pretty much useless. It's shot its wad, and all that's left is water on the floor. It's stopping that first wave from getting through that is the challenge. Once you've successfully done that, you can do something about making sure other waves stop coming.

In other words, once you turn the initial attack, you can do something about stopping him from attacking again. But if you don't get that initial attack turned, you're dog meat because he's NOT going to give you a chance to recover. The next attack is coming hot on the heels of the first one.[12] This is a major difference between the real thing and sparring.

When you can keep from being overwhelmed by such wave-like attacks in various situations then you can bring your art up and out and use it to defeat your attacker. This is where you go from being the whupee to doing some whuppin' yourself. (Or show your intelligence and beat feet!)

As I have said before, there is a whole lot more going on in a self-defense situation than just the moves. If you don't realize this, that's how Mr. Murphy will get you. It's easy to think that you know about these issues and have them under control. However, that's very much like someone fresh out of boot camp thinking that he is ready for the jungles. Wrong!

Having a plan of action in place in the event you're ambushed in an alley or some Neanderthal goes off on you in a bar is not the kind of thing people normally think about. With standard thinking, there's no way you could know these issues or recognize their significance. Unless you have been there or trained under someone who has tailored a system to address these issues, you're not going to find your way through that strange territory.

If you've never had to stand up against an all-out attack on the street, you need to seek out a scenario-based training course. I highly recommend established combat courses such as Model Mugging, IMPACT, Awakening the Warrior Within, or Rocky Mountain Combat Applications Training.[13] These courses usually serve as a serious wake-up call. Be warned, they are expensive. But they have been tailored over the years to prepare people for the mental and emotional stress of a real altercation. Unlike many local dojos that hold occasional self-defense workshops, these established groups have spent years studying the psychological issues involved. They have the cushions in place for the time your world gets tweaked. And believe me, tweaked it will be, even if you've been in the martial arts for years. These courses are the closest you can safely get to a live-fire situation. I cannot stress enough how much of an eye-opening experience it can be.

---

[1] A movie about what my smart-assed stepdaughter refers to as the "pterodactyl days." It's cinematic proof why, if you claim to remember the '70s, you weren't there.

[2] Murphy's Law: Whatever can go wrong will go wrong.

[3] I've seen perfect judo throws totally messed up by the guy who is being thrown going "EEK!" and grabbing onto the nearest thing around to keep from falling. Bad news is that the nearest thing just so happens to be the guy doing the throw. All of a sudden they both end up on the ground.

[4] There is some debate as to the proper spelling of armor. Not only among editors on either side of the pond, but between historians and military. I follow the train of thought that armour indicates the stuff the knights wore and rode around

in until their horses dropped dead. Armor is the modern mechanized stuff that you drive around in and blow things up with. While both are fun, only one is air-conditioned.

[5] Although it is important to realize the fight was intentionally taken there by a ground fighter. In doing so, he took the fight to where his strengths really worked.

[6] For those of you who say jeet kun do (JKD)—you just hit a personal sore spot with me. What's being called jeet kun do has been slowly mutating into a martial arts style. Jeet kun do as it was explained to me is NOT a fighting style! It's a philosophical approach to analyzing and thinking about the martial arts, fighting, and body mechanics. Much of what is being taught as jeet kun do is a mishmash of effective techniques from other styles, stuff that was brought in after Lee's death. What you see being sold as JKD—if it didn't have Lee's name and a lot of mumbo jumbo attached to it— would be called simple cross-training. Read the *Tao of Jeet Kun Do* and make your own assessment of what Lee meant. Don't buy other people's interpretations, especially when they tell you about things like "jeet kun do techniques" instead of concepts. From what I have seen, JKD is rapidly being locked into a mode, which in my opinion goes against what Lee was trying to break free of when he talked about the "way of no way."

[7] This was originally addressed in my first book on streetfighting, *Cheap Shots, Ambushes, and Other Lessons: A Down and Dirty Book on Streetfighting and Survival.* It was covered much more extensively there.

[8] I have both books and videos on surviving a trip to the floor in the real thing. If you're interested in knowing the difference, I recommend you read *Floor Fighting* and watch the video *Down, But Not Out.*

[9] As seen in his video *Self-Defense against the Sucker Puncher.*

[10] There is a concept in the Western world that a person resides not in his/her body as much as the head and shoulders. Forensics has shown us that you can look at a murder victim's body and often tell if the killer knew his victim.

Often killers who know their victim will attack the head and shoulders (as if to punish the victim), whereas strangers tend to go for the body

[11] Chris Caracci's *Hand to Hand Combat for the Patrol Officer* is a great video if you're in a profession where you might have to physically restrain someone. Not just cops, but prison guards, bouncers, security, hospital orderlies, etc., all would benefit from watching Chris's tape.

[12] I have seen many people block the first attack and then get taken out by the second or third. That's because they are so upset about the first one that they don't do anything to stop the next attack from coming. If you block an attack and get hairless about it, then that attack has succeeded. You not only have to stop the initial attack from landing, but do something about his ability to attack again. If you don't, he's going to keep on pounding on you until he gets through. And why not? You're just standing there.

[13] All of these can be found on the Web, and at least one will be conveniently located near wherever you are. Of course, looking in the back of this book might also help you out.

CHAPTER 5

Axes and Centerlines

....

What's mine is mine, and what's yours is mine.

—The philosophy of any 2-year-old

When people ask me what style I teach, I tell them "2-year-old kung fu." Our *kiyai* is "MINE!" That's because in any confrontation, we have the same determination as a 2-year-old for getting what we consider rightfully ours. And what we consider rightfully ours is the centerline—yours, ours, and everything in between. And once we get the centerline, you're in deep kim chee.[1]

Remember I said that we'd be coming at this subject from the viewpoint of principles? OK, here's a biggie: The human body moves in circles. In fact, we're kinda like a wheel, and the centerlines are our hubs. And that's why 2-year-old kung fu works so well; it grabs ahold of the other guy's hub! All of a sudden that thing that all of his motions are based on resides in your hot little hands! Wanna bet that's going to mess up his day, plus anything he's going to try to do to you?

I've seen all sorts of drawings to explain centerline, but the one I like best is this:

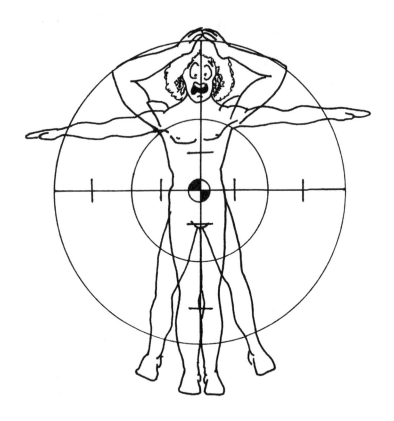

Leonardo da Vinci should be hitting turbo in his
grave about now for what I've done to his picture.
Still, it is probably the best explanation of what I'm
going to be talking about in this chapter. If you consider the cross hairs to be lines of a gyroscope, you
begin to see the axes of the human circle. Think
back to the geometry class (you know, the one

where you spent more time trying to see down the blouse of the girl who sat next to you than listening) and remember that an axis is the line around which a rotating body turns. Kinda like a planet's axis.

However, it also means "a central line bisecting a body, form, or the like, and in relation to which symmetry is determined."

If you're saying, "huh?" right about now, let me put it to you simply: It is around these imaginary lines the human body will spin—and spin the easiest!

These lines lead to the hub of the wheel. If you want to put what is here over there, what is up down, what is down up, these lines are where it will all happen. Want to put his head where his feet are? Use that horizontal axis. Put a hand up high, put a hand down low and push/pull so your hands trace

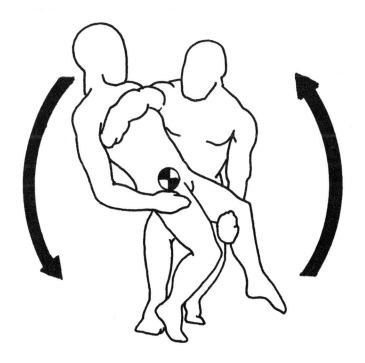

the circumference of his circle. His head and his feet also trace the circumference of that circle. Wheee!

We are designed to move around these lines. If we weren't, we'd stagger around like Frankenstein's monster. Because we're designed to move this way, we're designed to be unable to resist this way. While not exactly a design flaw, it is something you can exploit and use to your advantage.

One of these two centerlines is involved in almost every move you make with your body, whether you use it as a hub or a dividing line (or in the case of the horizontal one, a hinge). Well, guess what? That applies to your opponent, as well. These systems are always there and are vulnerable to your attacks. And you don't have to be a superman to use them, either.

Let me ask you a rhetorical question. Let's say you wanted to wreck an enemy's car with him in it. Is it easier to sabotage an existing system that controls the car—so your enemy drives it into a wall and totals the car—or is it easier to take a sledgehammer and demolish it with him inside it?

For those of you who said the first, congratulations. You see, it's easier to mess up an existing control system than it is to attempt to pummel a large object into the ground through raw force. Having established that, however, why in God's name do people insist on trying to end a fight by pounding someone into oblivion, instead of the much simpler way of tweaking the sucker and letting him nose dive into the concrete?[2]

Tell you what, let's make sure the sucker can't even control his body, much less get an attack aimed at you. It's hard to punch someone out when you are busy crashing into walls. Does this seem more reasonable to you? Good. Because that's exactly what getting ahold of his centerline is going to do for you.

My old sifu used to tell me that if a fight lasted longer than three moves, I was doing something wrong. He was right. Thing is, most people go into a fight with the wrong goal. They go in with the idea of winning or of pounding the guy until he's flat. While they're floundering around trying to make this squirrely idea work, who should show up but old Mr. Murphy.

Let me give you a new and improved goal here. Immediately after neutralizing the threat of any specific attack on you, your next move should be getting ahold of one of his centerlines. Oh sure, you could hit him six or seven times instead, but once you have ahold of a centerline, the sucker is a short second from slamming into the ground. And that means the end of the fight. I don't know about you, but that is a whole lot more appealing to me than waiting around for things to really go wrong.

Realistically, I can't expect you to be able to ditch years of training and just grab him like I can, but you seriously need to drop the idea that you're going to end a fight by just repeatedly hitting someone. If you really feel you must, go ahead and pop him one while you're reaching for the centerline and get it out of your system. But don't lose sight of your real goal of getting his centerline.

In case you haven't noticed, two guys punching each other is a fight, whereas one guy down and the other whomping on him is called a stomping. That's how most fights end. It's what he wants to do to you. Well, me hearties, you aren't going to let that happen. In fact, we're going to do unto him before he does unto you.

Well, not exactly what he's planning on doing to you, but close. See, he's planning on overwhelming you with his wave-like attack and crushing you to the ground. Trying to do the same would result in a clash—like two buffalo grunting, snorting, and pushing each other back and forth until one wins. Since that doesn't seem like an appealing idea, let's look at some alternatives.

One of the best ways to do this is to reach in and take control of his centerline. I'm not talking about necessarily grappling with the guy and wrestling him to the ground, although this does occasionally happen. What I am talking about is going in with the express intent of immediately gaining control of one of his centerlines and moving him around until he meets Mr. Gravity. This is messing up an existing system, and, as we all know, that's easier. Believe it or not, moving him so he meets gravity isn't a hard job, either. It's just a matter of moving him around his centerline.

What a lot of people don't realize is that you can get control of his centerline without getting that close to him. Sure, you can do it up close, but you can reach out and grab him, too! While details change, the principle of moving him around his centerline doesn't.

A really easy way to understand many throws is that they basically take the guy and make some part of his body trace his circle. (Head and feet trace the circle of the horizontal axis; shoulders and arms trace the vertical one.) You put your hands somewhere on either side of one of his axes, then push and/or pull, and whoopeeee! Around he goes.

The easiest way for you to make him go around his circle is for you go around yours. Yes, Ducky, in case you haven't realized it, your body works in circles too. Since this is the case, you might as well use it to your advantage.

Let me do a quick sidetrack here. Many people have difficulty with takedowns and throws. Part of the problem (as it has been expressed to me) is they

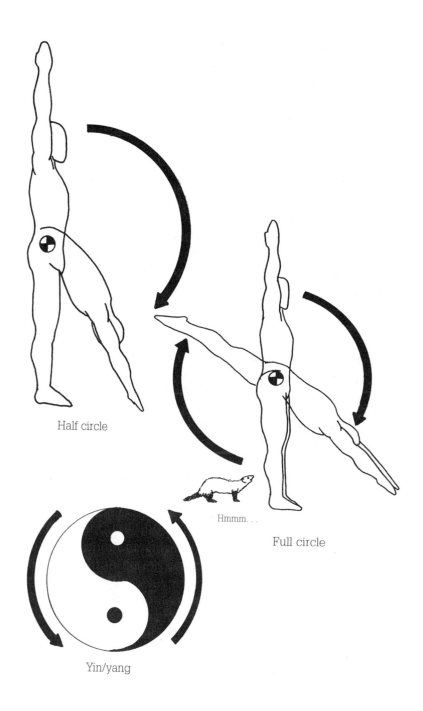

Half circle

Full circle

Hmmm...

Yin/yang

Axes and Centerlines

think they have to move in two directions at once. Let's fix that glitch right now. It might help if you stop thinking of it as moving in two directions at once and look at it for what it is—you moving around your own circle.

Most of the time we move in only a half circle. We're not accustomed to moving in the full circle, which is where the confusion comes in. Take a look.

By expanding how we move to encompass a full circle, we can remove all sorts of confusion. That full circle isn't going in two different directions any more than a spinning pencil on a desktop is going in two directions. Basically, it's either a clockwise or counterclockwise spin. The nature of a spinning circle is that as one side goes down, the other comes up. It's a yin/yang sort of thing.

When one side comes forward (pushes), the other side goes back (pulls)—but it is all done around that center axis. If you can stand in the middle of the room and spin around, you can move around your vertical axis. Or another real toughie to master—if you can walk, you're doing an abbreviated version around your horizontal one.

Both your body and his work this way. But what you're going to exploit as his weakness is going to be used as your strength. By knowing about the human circles, you gain strength, and he suffers. This is because there is incredible power in the torque created by a spinning object. Much of it rides on the circumference of the circle. And whatever it hits it will affect, as anyone who's tried to grab a spinning wheel will attest. Guess what you're going to be hitting him with? Riiiiight!

However, if you only use half circles, you're not going to have that power, and you'll need to resort to muscle to achieve your goals. That's why many people have a hard time learning throws and take-

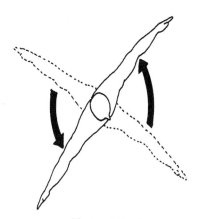

Horizontal spin

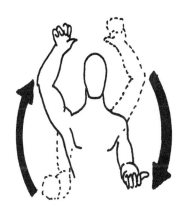

Vertical spin

downs—they're only moving half their bodies. They end up trying to use muscle because they aren't getting the power of the full circle. This is like throwing away a free steak and lobster dinner to eat macaroni and cheese.

You need to learn to use the full circle of your body—not just the upper half. It might help to imag-

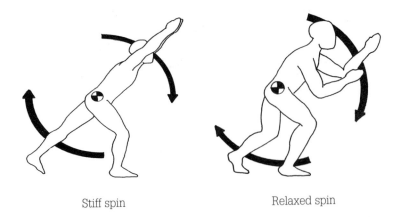

Stiff spin   Relaxed spin

ine you're moving inside a giant globe. It's not moving in two directions at once; it's rolling along.

Stay stiff until you understand the principle. Once you get the hang of it, loosen up. Start playing with all the different ways you can wiggle while moving around your circle. There is incredible power hidden within moving around your centerline.

After watching more judo, jujutsu, aikido, and yudo (the Korean form of judo) classes than I can shake a tonfa at, I can definitely state that the second most common problem people have doing throws is that most are not moving their opponent along the circumference of his body's circle.[3] They push in a straight line, not along his circle (or even theirs). Not only is it physically easier to move him along his circle, but it's physically harder for him to resist.

ANIMAL'S IMPORTANT SAFETY TIP

- It's easy to resist any force that is only going one way (i.e., pushing back or down). However, it's nearly impossible to resist a force that is pushing two direction at once (e.g., down and back at the same time). Our bodies are just not rigged for this kind of problem. If you shove or pull straight back or forward, he can resist you. However, when you push along the circle, you are pushing in two directions at once, back and down. When you are pulling along the circle, you are pulling in two directions at once, forward and up. If you don't follow the circle it will be a disaster.

The first technique will fail 90 percent of the time because the guy is being pushed backward, not backward and down. All he has to do is step back in order to make the shove ineffective and regain his balance. In other words, he's still standing and able to punch your lights out.

In the second illustration, however, the guy is not only being shoved back but DOWN! The guy doing the takedown is following the circumference of the other guy's circle as well as his own. This blows the sucker out of his cone of balance[4] and makes him fall down and go BOOM! It doesn't matter if he steps back to catch himself; he's still going to fall.

A useful training tip you should keep in mind is: Don't just send him off in a general direction somewhere over yonder. Point him where you want him to go. It's amazing how this little thing has such a profound effect on making sure he talks with the ants.

Look ma, no hands! Well, hands high, legs low. You can use both to get the guy flying. There's no law that says you can't use your legs to get a push/pull going against your opponent. In fact, it's part of your circle, so why not use it?

Whether you use your hands or your legs to do it, the principle is still the same. With a push/pull, you move the person around his horizontal axis, thereby spinning him around his circle. You get some poor slob stuck in this kind of shearing action and you're hitting him with four directions

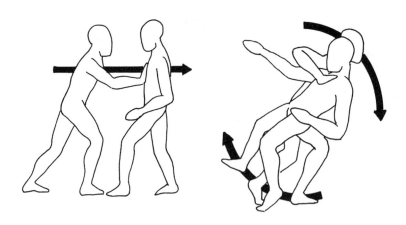

Shoving straight vs. following the circle

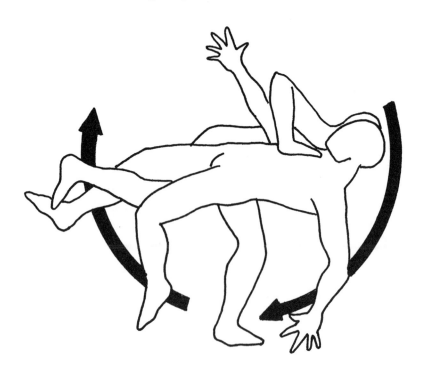

Taking It to the Street

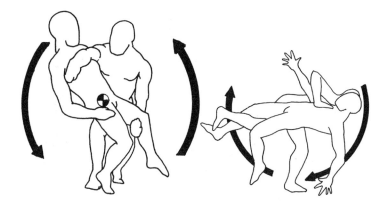

at once. Back and down, forward and up. I reckon
he's goin' down.

Keep in mind that the bigger you make the circle, the easier it is to move him. You can take
someone down with your hands less than a foot
apart on either side of that horizontal axis line, but
it's a lot of work. Two feet is still a chore, but
hands and legs apart 3 feet or more, and it's a
whole lot easier. That's because you're using
leverage more than muscle.[5]

This high/low split is one of the best ways to
take someone down. You'll see it in many a judo,
jujutsu, and aikido throw. Many Japanese grappling
stylists use their thighs or hips to establish the
lower point of control and put their arms across the
person's upper chest for the upper one. Once there,
wheeee! Many Filipino and Indonesian styles use a
combination of hands and feet to get a similar
push/pull action. These practitioners will hook your
ankle with theirs and pull it out from underneath
you while shoving your upper chest or grabbing
your face and shoving.

The important part isn't so much where or how
you grab him, but that, one way or the other, you

move him around this axis line. The axis, not the specific grab, is what makes the technique work.

ANIMAL'S IMPORTANT SAFETY TIP

- Here's an important safety tip we'll fully address later that's worth knowing now: There are more ways to attack with your feet than just kicking. In fact, some of the most effective foot attacks aren't kicks. If you learn how to use your feet offensively—without kicking—you will be able to defeat most opponents. Even someone who is a trained kicker will fall victim to this kind of foot-based offense. Since most people don't expect an ankle-level attack, they are REAL susceptible to it, especially if you pull their feet out from under them.

On a related topic, when you are attacking high/low like this, you don't have to put too much energy in the lower area. If you've ever tripped over a crack in the sidewalk, you know how little it takes to end up doing a nosedive. Just planting your foot in the right place can do the trick if your upper push/pull follows his circle. He's going to try to catch himself by stepping. But if your foot is in the way, all sorts of trouble will happen.

OK, back to messing up people's centerlines. One of the fastest ways to exploit the horizontal axis is to just grab the back of his head and fold him in half. Apparently, there is a great deal of confusion about how to do this very simple act. What we have here is what I call a "Bisquick scenario" (if it's too simple, people think they have to make it harder).[6] The truth is, taking someone down is really easy.

Guru Stevan Plinck[7] says, "Human beings are two-legged milking stools. The fastest and easiest way to take someone down is to put them where the third leg would be."

Bingo. That is the most exact, yet simple, way of explaining it I have ever heard. If you keep that simple rule in mind, you will know how to take him down no matter how he is standing. If he moves, fine, you'll still know how to drop him. The only thing that has changed is his position, not that there are two places for that third leg to be.

For those of you who are still a little hazy on this concept, try using a forward (and downward) jerk to put the guy's head between his knees. Not over a knee, but in between them. This folds him around his horizontal axis and puts him down where a third leg of the milking stool would be.

This is incredibly easy to do if the guy is swinging. He's given you the momentum that you need to mess him up. Remember the three-move limit? Here it is: block, grab the back of his head, and plant him.

While it is tempting to go out and try this move right now, there are things I will be discussing later in this book that will make it much more effective. Namely, you'll learn how to put your entire body weight behind this move so the poor slob literally has you dangling off his head. (Good luck resisting, Pal.) What is important now is that you get the idea of how easy it is to wrap someone around his centerline.

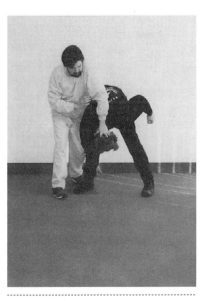

Head between the knees

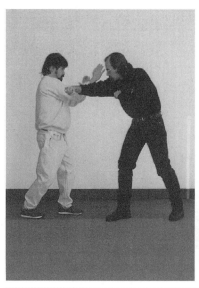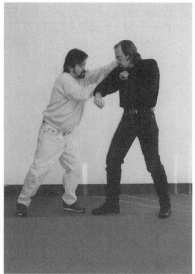

There is a very good reason I use the scoped drawings that first appear on page 82 to illustrate the importance of this point. Notice that through all of the illustrations, the guy has a little crash test dummy dot where the lines cross? That, mi amigos, is a thing called the center of balance, center of gravity, or center of mass. If you want to get esoteric, it's called his "one point" in some martial arts styles.

Well, like the name "T-post pounder," it pretty much tells what the thing is for. I like center of balance (or CB for short). It is the center of his balance and the center of his ability to stay upright, which means it is really vulnerable to attack (insert evil chuckle here).

So let's take a look at what we know about this sucker already: 1) It's on the horizontal axis, and 2) it's one of the major folding points of the human body. These are useful things in and of them-

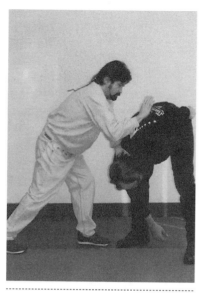

selves—but wait there's more! All of the guy's upper body weight is sitting on that giant hinge. But that weight is not sitting there like a lump of clay; it's always moving and shifting, as is the CB to stay under it. If for any reason that hinge gets knocked out from under his torso, or it can't get back under it in time, gravity takes over. My, my, my, isn't that interesting? If all of a sudden that structure holding up his weight were to go away, he'd come crashing down. That do present some opportunities, don't it?

Knocking the CB aside is the basis of more throws and takedowns than there are crooked politicians—in other words, a whole lot.

Until you break that line, his body weight is connected to the ground and under his control. Once you've knocked it out from underneath him, you can twist and contort him in all sorts of ways until he hits the ground. That's because a majority of his body weight is no longer anchored to the ground. He's flapping in the wind. From this point, you can spin, flip, bend, fold, spindle, or mutilate him as you will.

There are many ways to break the guy's center of gravity. Hands, hips, or knees—all can be used to blow it out from underneath him.

This is the secret of hip throws. Your hip is

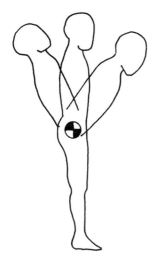

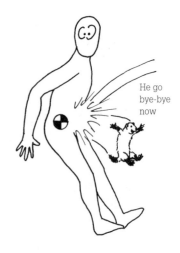

He go
bye-bye
now

Weight over center of balance   Center of balance knocked aside

doing the actual attack. It is swooping underneath
his and scooping up his center of gravity, thereby
blowing it out from underneath him. Once you've
done that, you move him so he can't regain it. Your
hands really aren't doing the throw. While they may
add some force to the process, their real purpose is
to keep him from recovering his balance and to
direct how he falls.

I'd like to add one more thing to the subject of
throws, and that is, simply, if you start to take someone down, make sure you throw him off you! As
soon as you get him moving around his centerline or
blow his balance, get him as far away from you as
possible. Throwing him off where you want him to
fall prevents him from grabbing on and taking you
with him. I'm not talking about tossing him off over
yonder; I mean, "I want you to fall right there!"
with a shove.

Taking It to the Street

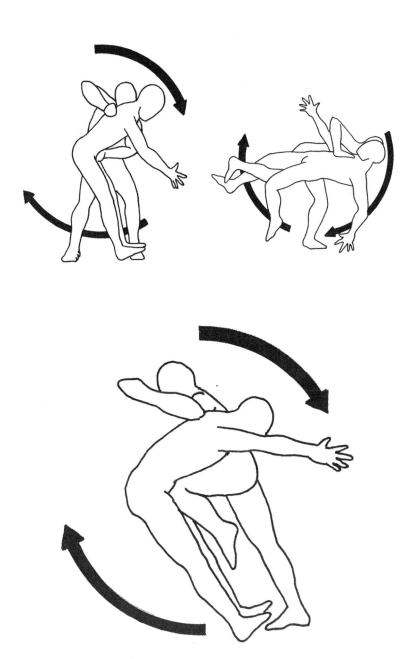

It's one thing to throw someone who's cooperating, but it's a whole 'nother issue to take someone down who is actively working against you. If you've ever competed in a grappling tournament, you know this. Stop and think of how many times you hit the mat hard because the guy was fighting you and somehow messed up your technique. Or somehow he managed to grab onto you and drag you down with him. Now imagine that same thing on concrete and landing on debris to boot—because that's exactly what is going to happen. Remember, he ain't on your side. Even if he doesn't intentionally counter your move, his flailing around can mess you up.

I'll tell you one of my favorite techniques for messing up a throw I can't escape. The best thing about it is that it just happens to be a natural reaction for someone who is falling. I try to grab onto the nearest thing to catch myself. Guess who's the nearest thing—YOU! Everybody is so impressed when they can turn their body weight and motion against their attacker that they forget that in one panic move he can do that exact thing right back to them![8] This is why it is so important to get him off you quick once you've blown his centerline (or CB). Here's a hint: Don't use muscle to get him moving, but use it to get him as far away from you as possible. Later on, you'll begin to see what I mean.

Now, if you want a really smoking explanation of how all of these principles work, go out and get Bob Orlando's book *Indonesian Fighting Fundamentals*. It's a great book, and Bob is very good at explaining these concepts in easy-to-understand terms like "shearing" and "gyroscopic rotation." (The latter sounds intimidating until you see the photo of him standing there with a bicycle wheel.) In the meantime, go out and play with these concepts to see how they can work with whatever style you know.

When you are going one way and your opponent is going the other, you're going to run into each other. I'm not talking arm's length running into each other while throwing punches. I'm talking cheek to jowl, hip to hip. You're throwing punches, and all of a sudden, BAM! You're clinched up. This happens a whole lot!

Does it mean that you immediately have to take it to the ground? No! In fact you want to do everything in your power to keep from going down to the ground with the guy! It's fine and dandy if he slams into the ground, but you keep your feet. This is why knowing how to blow someone's CB in all sorts of different ways is important. If you're clinched, do it with your hip. If it's close and getting closer, use your knee. If you still have time, use your hands. The important thing is blowing his balance before he can blow yours. I know I am harping on this, but you do not want to go down to the ground in a street fight!

Now, I've heard a lot of lip service from grapplers saying that their main goal is to put the other guy down while staying up themselves. Well, what they're saying and what they're doing in competition and what they are teaching others to do are not one and the same. I've seen too many grapplers shield up, take a few hits as they charge in, and tackle their opponent. And both end up on the ground.

I will be the first to admit that I get hard-core cranky about this subject, especially now that would-be grapplers are as common as fleas on a dog. But hard experience has taught me hard lessons in this field.

Reason No. 1 you don't want to go to the ground: There are concrete curbs, bottles, and tables that do not exist in either the dojo or the ring but do exist in the real world. This complicates falling. I've seen bottles break under people on the floor and cut the bejeezus out of them. Since you're rolling around on the floor too, you are just as vulnerable to getting cut as he is.

Reason No. 2: Trouble doesn't usually come alone. If you are in a one-on-one situation, rolling around on the floor with the guy is fine and dandy. Problem is, a guy looking for trouble seldom does it without at least one buddy there to back him up. Do you think they are going to stand around passively watching you choke their friend? Guess again, Kemo Sabe. While you're busy with one guy, his friend is going to take you out from behind. Often with something large—like a chair.

I've heard grappling instructors respond to this issue with statements of "Well, we have multiple opponent techniques." BULL! I want to know what fancy ground technique he's going to use when I pull his head back and drag a knife across his throat as he's choking out my partner. That is a street response to someone taking a friend down.[9] Want to know something? I'm humane—well, at least quick. In most situations like that, his friends would just blindside you with a beer bottle and then proceed to kick you to death.

This is over and above the problem of "study for five years, and I'll teach you how to fight multiple attackers from the ground." You don't have five years, you need something that works now! And what works now is not going to the ground![10]

While it may sound like I'm down on grappling, the truth is I'm not. In its time and place, it is absolutely devastating, and I highly recommend you study it to round out your repertoire.

What I am down on is two things. One is taking a perfectly good sports style and calling it street effective. This is a matter of focus. A majority of what is being taught is sport fighting, and while that is a legitimate and valuable focus, you have to do serious fieldstripping before you even think of taking it to the streets.

The second issue I get cranky about is coming into a fight with the expectation of taking it to the ground. Don't go into a fight with intentions of forcing it into one range because that ain't gonna happen. Keep in mind, grappling is a last ditch solution for when things go seriously wrong. Don't make it an integral part of your fighting strategy.

Train for what happens most, and you'll be able to handle most of what happens. From where I sit, one of the best styles to handle the clinching problem is judo. Fieldstripping is still necessary, but since they work from up close, it covers much of what will be occurring when a nongrappler clinches. The object is to get him off you, not go down with him.

Once you have this skill under your belt, look into jujutsu, sambo, BJJ, aikido, and wrestling to cover the rest of the grappling issue. But the first thing to do is close the holes in your defenses when someone suddenly bumps up against you. That way, you can put him on the ground and still be upright to deal with his buddies.

---

[1] Kim chee is Korean sauerkraut with an attitude. To start with, they stick it in a jar and bury it in the back yard for six months to ferment. The fact that they put enough garlic and chili pepper in it that you overlook the fact that you're eating rotten cabbage should give you an idea of what it's like. I personally love the stuff, but it is somewhat of an acquired taste.

[2] I guess it must be a sense of accomplishment thing. "I spent 10 years studying my butt off so I can do all this work and successfully sledgehammer my enemy and his car into the ground before he runs me over." OK, fine.

[3] The most common is that they try to do it from a deep-rooted, wide stance. Don't work that way, chitlins; ya gotta move your feet and step—no movement, no force, throw no work.

[4] Explained in mind-numbing detail in *A Professional's Guide to Ending Violence Quickly*. A quick summary: The cone of balance is the imaginary inverted cone we stay upright in. If we go beyond its boundaries, we fall down.

[5] If you want a good explanation of the forces you're going to be using with this stuff go out and get David MacAulay's book (or CD ROM), *The Way Things Work*. If you teach the martial arts, I really recommend you go out and get it. It's a great book, easy and fun, and it and makes explaining martial arts moves to your students a whole lot easier.

[6] According to my sweetie Dianna's old home economics teacher, years ago food manufacturers had the ability to make dried batter that only needed water added. However, housewives of the time felt that it was too simple and they weren't really cooking. The company changed the mix so you had to put in eggs, oil, and milk, which made the customers feel like they were really doing something.

[7] Steve's video, *Bukti Negra Pukulan Pentjak Silat* is one for which I set aside my standard "highly recommend" endorsement and put on a cheerleading dress and go "rah rah" over. It is fantastic. No matter what level you are at, you will learn from it.

[8] I take it a step farther and actually throw myself into the takedown. This removes the control of the throw, as well as dragging him with me.

[9] As an interesting point, I have heard from several different sources that there is a tendency in Brazil for people to stand back and watch a fight. Under those circumstances, it's relatively safe to go to the ground. However, that is not the case everywhere. In most places, people will jump in and help a friend. And even in places where it is supposed to be common, I'd hate to risk being the one that found the exception to the rule.

[10] Of course, scuttling like a crab underneath a nearby table or up the leg of a bystander has a long and proven track record for surviving trips to the floor in the real thing.

Centerline

··

*Any complicated system that works is
based on a simple system that works—and
often the simple system works better.*
—The Tomb of the Unknown
Software Programmer

While it's good on the horizontal axis, 2-year-old kung fu really comes into its power with the vertical axis. In styles that use it, this is popularly called centerline. For those of you from styles that don't use it—you're about to have a religious experience. Once you get ahold of it, what you can do to someone is only limited by your imagination. Personally, I've got a reeaaally big imagination, and the more you play with yours, the bigger it is going to get, too. Not only is this centerline the axis of his vertical circle, it is also one of the best ways to attack, disorient your opponent, and defend against his attack. All these neat things rolled into one.

Before we go into all the cool things you can do with it offensively and defensively, let's take this concept 3-D. Imagine our dummy ticked off someone who works in a lumberyard. To show his appre-

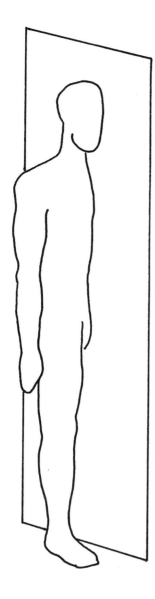

ciation, the guy stuck a hunk of plywood smack dab into our dummy's centerline.

The centerline extends outward. His vertical axis is a point on this line. From now on when I say centerline, I'm referring to this outward extension. When I say vertical axis, I'm talking about the pivot. Although they are one and the same (and that's how you need to start thinking about it), it should help clarify which aspect I'm talking about at a particular moment.

This centerline is not fixed in the middle of your sternum. It can extend outward in whatever direction you're facing. In fact, draw the centerline out in whatever direction your nose is pointing. No matter how you're standing, that's the outward manifestation of your centerline. That line comes in, connects with your vertical axis, and keeps on going. As all roads lead to Rome; all lines lead to the vertical axis.

Which is faster? Going in a straight line or going a roundabout way? Unless you're dealing with Los Angeles traffic, the answer should be "a straight line."

Next question: What is the shortest distance between two points? Again, straight line.[1]

Taking It to the Street

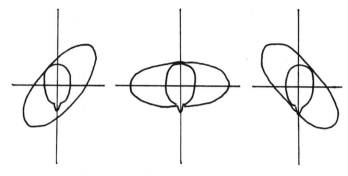

Centerlines

What is that extended centerline coming out from you? A straight line.

What is the extended centerline coming out from him? A straight line.

A whole lot of interesting stuff all comes back to this centerline issue. It's the shortest, fastest, and most effective way to get somewhere. If you become like a 2-year-old and refuse to share that centerline, what do you have? The fastest way to do something.

I first learned about the centerline in wing chun gung fu. Kali uses it, as well. When I got to silat, its use took off in a totally different direction.[2] Each of these styles uses this concept with devastating effectiveness. And once you understand it, you can have some serious fun with it. What I am going to tell you here is a total mishmash. It has its roots in all of these styles and more, but it is not pure any-thing. I did what I always do and fieldstripped these styles for application in the street. So I can't claim (nor will I) that it is any particular style or form. I would, however, recommend you go out and take a few seminars from those who teach the pure styles because the stuff is great, no matter what the focus.

OK, let's start out working on the defensive aspect. First, put your hands on the centerline.

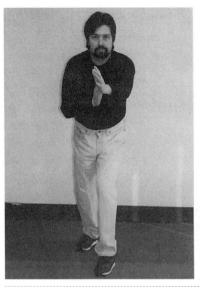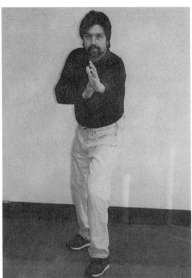

Centerline stances

Now what do these stances have in common?

The answer is each of them takes the centerline. (It's MINE!) Taking it to this level has one incredible advantage—it simplifies everything. I really like Bob Orlando's summation of what comes from this concept. In fact, I'm using his words. From the centerline there are only two ways to block. Block left, block right.[3] That's it. If you divide your body down the centerline, every block you do is to one side or the other. That's because every attack has to come in on either side of the centerline. It's real simple.

If you open yourself up, however, the blow can come in anywhere. Now instead of two ways, you have three potential ways for a blow to come in. Left, right, and up the middle.

What does your juvenile attitude about centerline do to anyone else's punch? It makes it go the long way around! *That means it's going to be slower*—even if he gets the jump on you with a punch. If

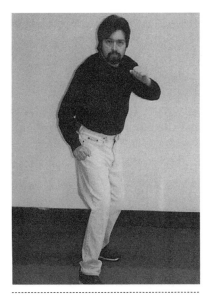

Open centerline stance—no, no, bad, bad!

you have your center-line, his punch has to go the longer route to get to you. It's going to take him a second longer to get there, which gives you a second more to react. Speaking of reaction time, let me tell you something that will keep you from getting your nose driven through the back of your skull. Recently, I sparred with a 21-year-old who has three black belts and speed that would make a rattlesnake gulp in disbelief. Here I am, an old man, fat, out of shape, who's nowhere near as fast as this kid. It was open sparring—no judges, no points, no time limit, and no stopping after a strike. It was the classic young buck against the old master kind of thing. Well, clichés get that way for a reason. The kid never touched me.

He's faster than me. He's stronger than me. He's a much better kicker. He's an experienced tournament fighter—in fact, he's a three-time state champion. Face it, he's your basic nightmare. Still he couldn't connect.

Why?

Aside from the fact that I had my centerline (and every time he tried to take it, he got jack-slapped), the other reason was I always saw him coming. That is to say, every time he threw a punch or a kick, by the time it got there—I was waiting for it.

How could I do this if he's faster than I am? It was because I wasn't watching his hands or feet—those were too fast for these tired old eyes to follow.[4] I was, instead, watching the source of his blows, and that is where I was blocking.

Let's take a quick trip back to that geography class we were talking about earlier . . . oh no, wait, the geography part was checking out the landscape next to you. It was a math class. Anyway, remember that little tidbit about the circumference of a wheel traveling at a higher speed than the hub? Even though they travel the same number of degrees, a point along the circumference has to travel faster because it has to cover more distance (out on the circumference, the points are farther apart). So, just plucking numbers out of the air—knowing that they are totally wrong—the hub is moving at 5 mph while the same point out on the circumference is moving at 15 mph.[5]

Realize, however, that even though the outside point is moving faster, the hub starts moving at the same time. By watching the slower hub, you can easily predict where the faster point will be coming in and, more importantly, keep it from getting there!

The fist traces the circumference of a hook, but the top of the arm/shoulder is the hub. The fist could be anywhere and coming in from any direction, but I guarantee you it's going to be attached to the guy's shoulder. By watching the hub instead of trying to watch the fist, you can see the attack coming before it gets to you. And that gives you time to do something about it.

Let me give you a good analogy. Your opponent's fist is like a missile. Once he launches that missile, it's really hard to shoot it out of the sky. But that is exactly what most blocks are trying to do—catch the sucker in mid-flight before it lands. What if, instead

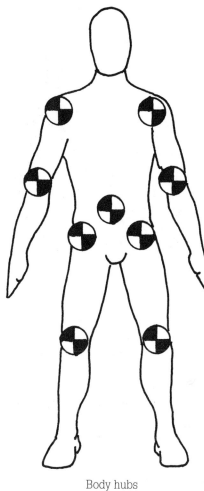

Body hubs

of watching your own airspace and frantically trying to catch missiles as they come speeding into it, you watch his missile's launch pad? It's easier to scrub the missile as it launches than it is to knock it out of the air. You know where it's going to be coming from, so that's what you focus your attention on.

While my eyes can't keep up with the speed of that fist, they can track movement in the shoulder and upper arm! The moment I see those parts move I know something is coming! And that is where I am going to aim my counterattack to scrub the missile during its launch! This is, by the way, one of the main secrets of counterpunching.

The hubs of his attacks are the shoulders and the hips. When they move in a "just-so" way, an attack is being launched! I cannot accurately describe it in a book, but most often it is a

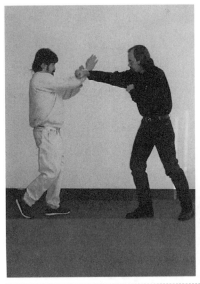
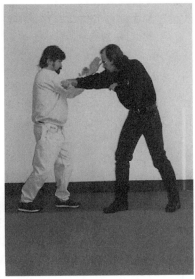

Shallow block (no)   Deep block (yes)

"rising/rolling" action. It's kind of like a reversed rowing-a-boat action in the shoulder. Spend a few weeks watching televised boxing matches and other people sparring. After a while, this shoulder roll will become blatantly obvious to you.

Once you have gotten to the point where you can spot it, sit with your hands in your lap. Mirror the guy throwing the punches by patting your thighs. When you see the shoulder roll, tap your hand on the same side. From there, it is a tiny step to just shooting your hand out for a block. Your goal with this block is to reach as far in as you can to that hub and mess up the missile's launch at the shoulder.

If you know where to look and what the signs are, an opponent will tell you what he's about to do. Do the math. If his right shoulder is moving toward you, odds are the attack is going to come from the right! To further refine this, if that shoulder is drawing back, which quadrant is the attack going to be coming from?

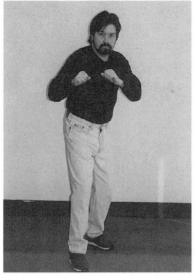
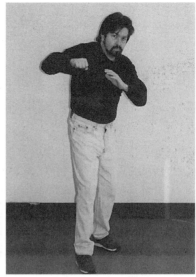

Boxing jab, beginning,   middle,

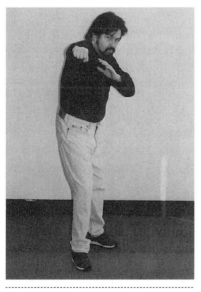

and end

The upper left! Where does it suddenly make a whole lot of sense to get a hand up to?

We'll go more into elbows and knees later. But let me tell you right now, they will tell you what is coming the second the guy launches his attack!

The key element is his elbow's location in relation to his shoulder and centerline. Since they are connected with a straight

line (it's called an upper arm), this is easy to figure
out. If the elbow is high, the attack is coming in
high on that side; if it's low, then it's coming in low
on that side.

When his knee is up in the air, the attack will
come from the same side of the centerline it's on. If
his knee crosses the centerline, you can bet dollars
to doughnuts that he's going to try to lay some sort
of back hook, ax, or crescent kick from that new side
on you. But if he plants that foot and sets it down on
that new side, he's going to spin on you. Which side
will he be coming at you from when he spins? The
same one as before. Go out and watch for these patterns, and you'll begin to see them as plain as day.
And once you begin to see them, it becomes really
easy to foil attacks.

SIMPLIFYING A BRAWL

Here's something that should make this all a little bit less scary. Granted, it's a simplification, but
realize that for the moment it takes him to attack,
you don't have to worry about anything else. One
attack is all you have to deal with at that precise
moment, even if it's a fake or blindingly fast.
Because, simply stated, few people attack in more
than one place at once. They are simply not trained
to launch multiple attacks. Even someone who is
chaining his attacks is following a one-two-three
pattern. It's one attack at a time.[6]

It's incredible how much it will help to take this
simple statement to heart. You don't have to worry
or fret about where the attack is coming from. You
know where it's coming from—RIGHT THERE!
That's all he's doing at this moment, and stopping it
is all you have to worry about at this moment. The
second his hand starts retreating back, that attack is

over. Whatever happens next, you deal with it when it happens.

That wavelike, blitzkrieg attack is the same thing. The guy is coming at you like a piston, one-two-three. This often means he's really attacking in one place. Personally, I love bozos like that. If he's not smart enough to figure out that pounding on only one place like a woodpecker on a battleship isn't working, he's also not bright enough to realize that while he's busy attacking with his right side, his unprotected left side is flapping in the breeze.

Simplification No. 1

This one-two-three pattern even applies to trained fighters. A good fighter comes in from different directions, one strike after another, which makes it seem like the guy is all over everywhere. The guy may be motherin' fast, but if you watch you'll see his attacks are sequential. What's confusing is the unexpected change of direction. Well, we've already solved half of that problem by taking the centerline. Which way is it going to come in from? Either left or right.

Simplification No. 2

Few people are trained well enough to have their attack blocked and immediately flow into another attack with the same movement. I'm not talking about a feint; I'm talking about a real dedicated attack that changes into something else when you block it. (A good example is a punch that folds into an elbow strike when blocked.) Most people either try to continue plowing forward with their ruined attack—which means it's still the same attack—or pull back and launch another attack. It may be lightning fast, but that sequential pattern is still there.[7]

Simplification No. 3

If his right side (not just his right arm) goes back, then automatically his left comes forward. Think maybe a trained fighter might use this to throw confusing blows that seem to come in from all sides? In fact, it's usually right, left, right. But, if he leaves that side out, odds are the next attack will come from there (jab, jab, jab).

So the only thing you have to worry about is dealing with that one attack, not what he's planning on doing next! Because if you derail his attack—not just block, but derail—you're also going to put his other plans in the mud! Who cares that he has this great combo attack planned to kick your butt, HE AIN'T GONNA GET A CHANCE TO USE IT![8]

Breaking down a fight to this time schedule will help you immensely. Instead of one giant, wild ball of chaos, you take it down into bite-sized bits that you can chew and digest. Let's say the whole fight may last only a minute. Ten different things may happen in that minute. If you're looking at it from the schedule of a minute, what you see is a totally incomprehensible free-for-all. However, if you look at the same minute in six-second chunks, you'll begin to see the sequential patterns I'm talking about instead of a wild furball.

Simplifying it to this level also means you react faster! When you do that, you're the most effective! It removes the "whadda I do?" confusion that messes up so many people in the real thing. Having all sorts of tools doesn't help you if you can't figure out which one to use.

There's an Aesop's fable about this very problem that might help you understand why simplification is important. A cat and a fox were talking about how they escaped from dogs. The fox bragged, "I have 10,000 ways to escape dogs." The cat said, "I have only one, I run up a tree." As they were talking, a dog charged out of the bushes. The cat immediately ran up the tree. The fox—while he was trying to decide which of his 10,000 techniques to use—was caught and torn apart.

The cat had a simple solution that he could enact immediately—that's why he survived. If the fox could have chosen which of the 10,000 would have worked best as quickly as the cat, he might have lived to brag some more. This is a problem facing many martial artists. What do you do to handle a charging dog? Simplification allows you to choose as fast as the cat.

Let's do some math here. Which of the 10,000 techniques that you know do you use to keep from getting hit by a right punch? Let's winnow them out. He's not coming down the centerline because you have it. That rules out a few techniques right there. He's swinging his right, which means it's coming in on your left. Any technique that doesn't constitute blocking/checking left is dropped faster than a pissed-off scorpion. That just cleared the deck of about 9,975 things to think about. Coming up and off centerline (which is a natural reaction, by the way) just cleared out another 20. Now it's your choice of what five things to do. One of them is going to appear to be the best bet immediately.

Boom! There's your answer. Your one way of escaping the dog just became clear. There's no confusion to make you hesitate like the fox. Whadda I do? You don't get hit: It's coming from your left, so you block left. Next question? Give it some time and practice and you'll be amazed how confident you become on this issue. "Yeah, yeah, I got your attack from the left right here . . . "

While we'll cover dealing with kickers later, the same thing can be said for spotting a kick coming at you. THE KICK WILL ALWAYS COME FROM THE LIGHT FOOT! Before he can kick, he *has* to shift his body weight off that foot! Gravity dictates that it is physically impossible to buck this rule. His center of balance will move over the supporting leg.[9] When the guy shifts his weight onto one leg or the other, he is telling you which side the kick will be coming from. That shift in his CB is a "just-so" movement. Learn to watch for it.

Tying this all back, take your centerline and extend it until it digs into his vertical axis and keeps going out behind him. I'm talking about using your mind to aggressively reach out and plant it into the clown. All of that and everything behind it to the horizon is yours. That is what owning centerline means.

Do this and, to quote my favorite asthmatic, "I have you now . . . " If he shifts his center of balance, if he wiggles, if he moves a hub, if he rotates around his axis, if he even burps . . . you'll know about it. You'll know what's coming long before it would ever be effective. By the time his attack gets to a place where it might have a chance, you'll already be there with a counter. "Bzzzzt, thank you for playing. Better luck next time."

The trick isn't being faster; it's knowing what he's up to quicker than he expects. He expects you to catch on to what he's doing when he clobbers you. Personally, I don't like that schedule. To keep from getting punched, you just move the schedule up a bit—like knowing what he's trying about the same time he does. That means your counter starts at the same time. It travels across town and is there waiting to meet him before he even gets close to you. "Gosh, that didn't work out at all the way you expected, did it, fella?"

Practicing what I've just told you can compensate for all sorts of issues regarding speed, reflexes,

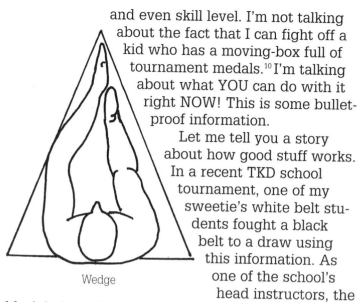

Wedge

and even skill level. I'm not talking about the fact that I can fight off a kid who has a moving-box full of tournament medals.[10] I'm talking about what YOU can do with it right NOW! This is some bullet-proof information.

Let me tell you a story about how good stuff works. In a recent TKD school tournament, one of my sweetie's white belt students fought a black belt to a draw using this information. As one of the school's head instructors, the black belt walked onto the mat thinking he'd play around for a bit then take our guy out. Next thing he knew, he was into it up to his ears. With less than two months of training and this information, our white belt managed a tie. So think what you could do with it.

Now let's address the most common defensive question about centerline that I hear: "What about circular attacks?" What about 'em? If you got centerline, we can sort of automatically assume that the guy is going to have to resort to hooks. The answer to both straight and circular attacks is in the elbows. Ever heard of jug-eared? Well you get to go jug-elbowed. In other words, they stick out like a taxi's doors.

Did you notice what shape is formed out in front? It's a triangle. Actually, it's probably better if you think of it as a wedge. If you've ever split wood with either a wedge and mallet or an ax, you know how effective a wedge can be. Whatever he

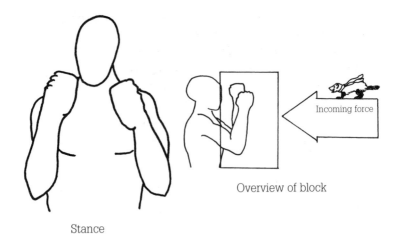

Overview of block

Stance

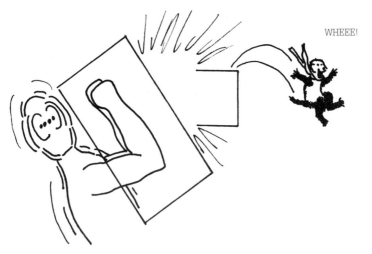

WHEEE!

Energy hitting block

throws is going to either deflect off or slam into the side of the wedge! This includes the sudden blitzkrieg attack.

Let's look at the straight shot first. Above you see a classic fighting stance. First thing to see about this stance is that really big, neat hole that it leaves open for your attacks along the centerline—but that's for later. The second thing is to consider what shape it creates in front of the fighter. The answer is a semi-solid block. Now answer me this, chitlins: What does an incoming force do when it hits a block?

If your answer was "BOOM! OW!" you are correct. All of that force is delivered. Some of it may be deflected, but most of it lands to ring your chimes. Even if you don't get hit, the block that you have out in front of you gets clobbered and it passes on to you. If you've ever held the kickbag when someone plants a shin kick, you know exactly of what I speak. This is all assuming that your blocking arm doesn't just fold up from the impact.

Now let's look at what happens with a wedge. That same straight, incoming force is deflected.

Even though there is some impact, the main force of the blow is deflected. That's just the very nature of the wedge. When you add a block or other motion to this equation, it becomes even more effective at deflecting the force.

The illustration below pretty much shows you what happens if the blow is coming in close to the centerline. But what happens if it comes in from a little farther out?

The answer is: nothing. Raise or lower your arm. The blow just lands on a different part of the wedge and deflects. Even a hook slams into the side of the wedge. If you get your elbow up (which

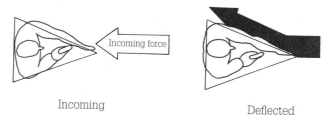

Incoming   Deflected

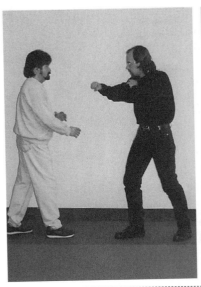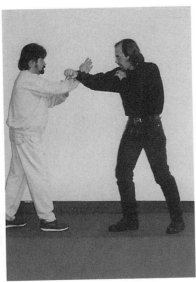

by reaching up and toward his hub, you're going to do anyway), his forearm slams into the wedge. It ain't going to get to you.

Raising your arm to cover up is the most basic of all blocks. It's also an instinctive reaction when someone is coming at you. The trick is to just do a natural reaction, modifying it so your hands come up and shoot out along the centerline. If your

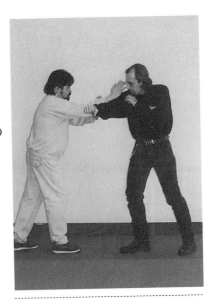

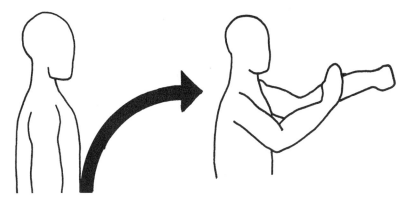

Shoot wedge

hands aren't on that centerline, just lifting your arm leaves major holes.

By lifting your arm in a wedge with at least one hand on the centerline, you create a barrier against your attacker. His attack must encounter that barri-

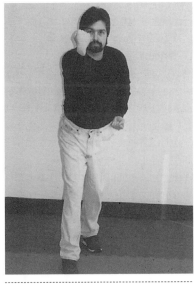

Karate block

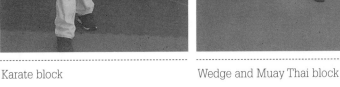

Wedge and Muay Thai block

er if you are even close to the right level.[11] But if you leave the centerline, what you're doing is sticking up two windshield wipers that you're hoping will stop an attack.

One of the most common problems I have seen is people's hands floating wide when they're under stress, especially against the blitzkrieg attack. This is what I was talking about when I said people chase attacks out to Outer Mongolia. They think by spreading themselves wide they protect themselves. This is not true; they create bigger holes by leaving the centerline. Trust the wedge. It protects you on many fronts. It keeps you on the centerline. If you lose the wedge, you lose the centerline. Giving up your centerline leaves you wide open for all sorts of things to come crawling up it or around it. Make his attack come to the wedge, not to a block of Swiss cheese.[12]

The same protection can be gained by shooting your hand out along the centerline. You mirror the side the attack is coming from. Remember block left, block right? If it's coming in from a certain side, that's the side you want to shoot out toward his missile launch pad. Notice at the same time that just scooting out along your centerline also automatically raises your elbow and arm, which traces back to the most basic block. This trick is really useful because it allows you to reach out and affect his hub, which we'll get into later.

Notice that in each of these photos, the elbow is still held out slightly catty-wompus. That keeps the integrity of your wedge, which is a foundation for not getting thumped.

Realize that from this centerline position, your hands don't have to move far to block. In fact, all you have to do is spin your elbow. Remember, it too is a hub.

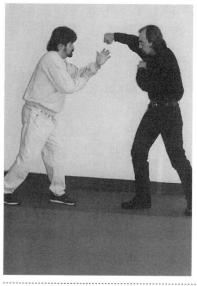
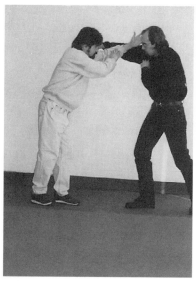

Centerline extended   Centerline extended more

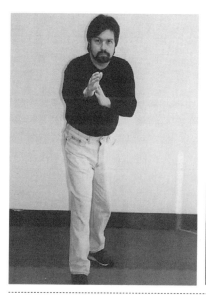
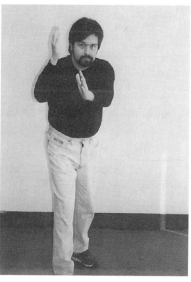

Blocking from the centerline

Centerline   127

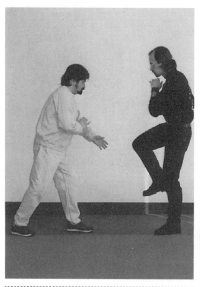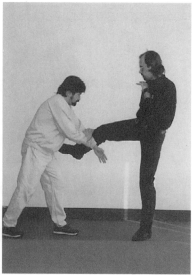

Low wedge against a kick

What I want you to realize here is that this gesture is now less of a block and more of a wipe-away. Shooting the wedge out into his face is the real block. This other action is more of a sweeping gesture that opens him wide up. It gives you a plethora of options, from grabbing him and jerking him down to opening up his defenses to snaking in an attack to spinning him to the side, etc.

This concept of keeping the centerline also works real well against kicks. Granted, if the guy is attacking you with his hands, you want to keep yours up. But if he decides to attack low, you can drop your wedge to meet the attack.

Even though the wedge works best when your hands are together, it also can work with your hands moving independently—as long as the shape of the wedge is maintained.

If you're not sure how the guy is going to attack, split the difference. You're still maintaining

Taking It to the Street

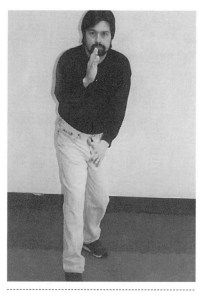

High-low split

the wedge and keeping the centerline. It might help you to understand this if you take a stick and lay it across the inside of your elbows. No matter which hand is high or low, by looking down at your arms you will see the triangle. Do it in front of a mirror, too. Even if your hands aren't on the same level, the integrity of the wedge and your control of the centerline are maintained.

I'd like to address something that seems to confuse many people who come from linear styles. You *can* leave the centerline with your front hand without giving up the centerline. Remember, this is 2-year-old kung fu. Just because you left it lying there in the middle of the floor doesn't mean it is no longer yours.

First off, if your front hand leaves the centerline for whatever reason, your rear hand comes forward to reclaim what is rightfully yours. This is usually a simultaneous action.

The real nasty application of this will become obvious in the offense aspect later on in this book. But for right now, practice shooting your hands out, your lead hand wiping away and your rear hand shooting forward.

But let's say that for some reason you opt not to shoot your back hand out. Your lead hand wipes

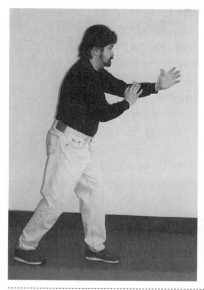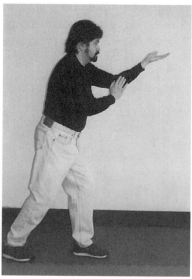

Choo-choo train

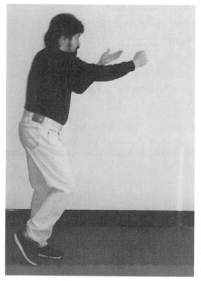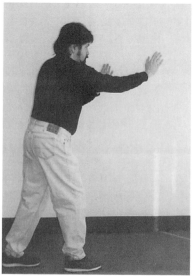

Taking It to the Street

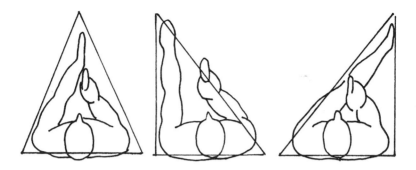

Triangles

away the blow. In doing this, you still maintain a triangle out in front of you. Take a look at the illustrations below.

I'm using only the left hand lead for illustration purposes, but I want you to realize you can do the exact same thing with either hand. In blocking either direction, you simply change from an isosceles triangle (ready position) to a right angle triangle (either block). The integrity of the wedge is still out in front, protecting you. All the while, that rear hand is back there waiting to shoot out over your other arm.

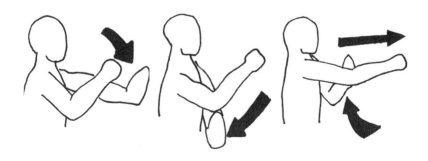

Block left   Return block   Return

For those of you who are saying, "Wait a minute, my sensei told us never to cross our arms," let me point out that I personally love it when people say that. Such a provincial attitude is why many a martial artist's centerline is always open for nasty people like me to exploit. In the blocking chapter, I will give you a critical bit of information about how to make this move work, but you will have to go out and work with it on your own to see if it works for you.[13]

One more point: Most martial artists fight for a centerline that is somewhere around a foot wide. Maybe they trim it down to a fist's width. Those hard stylists that are taught about centerline tend to fight for it head to head, believing it takes up a huge space.

Triangle centerline is pinpoint. You take centerline not by a foot but by millimeters.

When you hone this concept down to such a fine point, even if a blow is coming in along your centerline (or that sidewalk that most call centerline), you'll be able to manipulate it to the left or to the right, often with just your fingertips! When your centerline is that tiny, your fingertips may leave it but your wrists won't. Your fingers snake around his arm, and then your wrists slam into him and block either left or right.

Imagine your hands are wet rags. When you shoot your arms up, your hands flop around his forearm. That action gives your wedge block extra power, as well as putting them in a perfect place to do all sort of nasty things to him.

There are many things that you can do with this concept of the centerline. But the neatest of them all is that once you get the hang of using both hands on the centerline, someone trying to get through to punch you is going to have a real bear of a time. If you sit down and look at most fighting stances, they

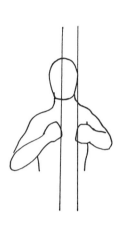

Wide centerline

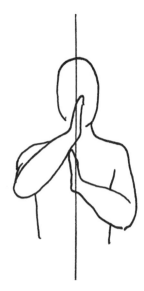

Thin centerline

only offer one thin line of defense over a particular area. Once that line is breached or bypassed—as often happens with a wave attack—then it's an open shot to the body. By putting your hands up like this and keeping centerline, you can put hands, arms, or elbows all over everywhere to keep that attack from ever touching you. If they can't touch you, they can't hurt you.

---

[1] Although some can convincingly argue that a tight blouse also qualifies, we won't go there.

[2] For those of you who say, "Hey! That's jeet kun do," yeah, it's a parallel path, including my study of philosophy and Eastern religions. However, years ago when I was a young street punk dodging knives and bullets for my indiscretions, I copped a real attitude with the Cult of St. Bruce. My wing chun sifu shared an academy with the main source of JKD

on Venice Blvd. There were more than a few "JKD True Believers" running around, and I had run-ins with some of them outside of the school. It's hard to stomach someone whose convinced he's some sort of invincible warrior when the weekend before you were crashing into walls with a pissed-off biker trying to eat your face. While I never started anything with any of them, in the same breath, apparently they weren't convinced enough of their style's invincibility to swing on me first. So it always stayed at the attitude stage (which was cool, because I was still sore from that biker incident). I have a friend who currently studies JKD, and he claims never to have seen any of this kind of behavior or superiority complex. Maybe it was just a tendency of that particular generation (and I freely admit, back then I was a real piece of work, too), but that was my experience—and it soured me on JKD.

The thing is I don't have a problem with what Bruce Lee said. Although I resisted reading *The Tao of Jeet Kun Do*, when I finally sat down and read it, I agreed with it. What he did was vital to organizing the martial arts for Western comprehension. In fact, I highly recommend you read it.

[3] Books and videos that I HIGHLY recommend you save your rupees and get are Bob Orlando's stuff on Indonesian fighting arts. The man is great at describing things in easy-to-understand terms.

[4] The sucker's feet are also too fast for young eyes to follow. They're a blur, and then there's this flash of light as he thumps you. Not fun at all.

[5] I asked a scientist buddy of mine for the exact equation. The simple answer he gave me was $V\_r = 2*pi*f*r$. The more complicated explanation nearly melted my brain. I think Randy gets great pleasure out of confusing me.

[6] It's the difference between a shotgun and an automatic pistol. With a shotgun loaded with 00 buck, one pull of the trigger launches the equivalent of nine 9mm slugs. That's multiple attacks—even if one misses, the others will get you. With an auto pistol, you have to pull the trigger nine times. Which one takes longer?

[7] This also includes feints, fakes, and Set Ups that are

designed to draw you in one direction while the real attack will be coming in from elsewhere. The way to handle that is don't go chasing attacks. There is no need to go running off to Outer Mongolia to block. If an attack is legit, it will come to you. There is no need to reach out to the side to block. The only reaching you need to do is forward, toward his missile base.

8   Again I have to to say that there are some extremely well-trained fighters out there who not only simultaneously attack, but attack on multiple levels. An example of this kind of attack is the guy who comes in with a blow at the same time he stomps on your foot. Like I said, though, this kind of problem is extremely rare, and you have to have been doing something seriously wrong to end up in these kinds of situations.

9   Or he'll jump, thereby giving up balance, support, mobility, and common sense. But that move is so suicidal in a real fight that I won't even bother addressing it. I will, however, point out that the time you really have to worry about flying kicks is against a trained fighter (or someone just flailing around) when you've taken him off his feet with a throw. As he's going down, he twists and whomps you one. It really rains on your parade to get your teeth kicked in as you're doing a great jujutsu move on the dude (which is what he intended on doing). This is why you always need to keep your guard up, even as he's going down.

10 Of course, the Three Stooges imitations also sort of helped to throw him off kilter, too. He finally lost it when he was in his fighting stance and I reached out and shook his lead hand and said, "How ya doin?" Who says I have to take this stuff seriously?

11 It kind of helps if you block high attacks high and low attacks low.

12 I will tell you this now: If you get hit from the front while using this technique in a sparring match, check your centerline. I'll bet you dollars to doughnuts that your hands have floated apart. When this happens, you give up your centerline and allow all sorts of nasty stuff to come creeping up it, including kicks to the face. Wide-open blocking positions work best against someone whose attacks are primarily cir-

cular (i.e., roundhouses and shin kicks) but suck against linear or hooking attacks

[13] Oh yeah, when I say go out and experiment with a concept, I don't mean go out and tell the ranking black belt what you're doing, and then let him rip you (and these concepts) to shreds. Especially if you study someplace where the attitude is "our way is the only way." NIH (Not Invented Here) is a serious problem in Westernized martial arts. If you tell such an instructor what you're working on, he's going to immediately rip it apart—and being forewarned, he'll probably figure out a way how. You're not advanced enough, yet. But if you just spring it on him or other students and see them confused by it, you'll see how well it works. After you've proven to yourself that it works, *then* take it to your teacher for review.

Blocking

Before I have to hit him
I hope he's got the sense to run.

—Grateful Dead
"Alabama Getaway"

What I want to do now is put the finishing touches on the defensive aspects of coming off the centerline. First, I want you to realize that your arms should not be tight and locked down when they are heading out there. Tight muscles may be powerful, but they are not fast. (Actually they're neither, but we'll go into that in a bit.) That means you get hit more because you can't get where you need to be in time to block his attack. Not good at all.

Instead of tight, hard tree branches, your arms need to be like two snakes. You know what I'm talking about if you've ever handled any kind of constricting snake. Boas can go from a soft touch on your hand to a bone-crushing force in a split second. But once the reason for being tense is past, they go soft again. By being soft, they are motherin' fast when they strike. By suddenly clamping down when they get there, they get back all the power they set aside for speed. If you're into evil entertainment, then you're going to love this one. Those hard, tree-branch arms of your opponent are exactly what your snakes are going use to slither along to get to his tender spots. It may not seem like it at first, but this snake-arm stuff is a brutal and nasty combination.

Here's a series of exercises I want you to try:

Phase one: Stand up. Now relax the muscles in your arms. Let them dangle. Then start quickly tensing and relaxing them. Something you need to pay close attention to is relaxing as fast as you tensed. It's not a matter of tightening and then gradually letting go. You stop tensing just as quickly as you started. Now comes the tricky part. Start doing just your forearms, then your upper arms. When you do this, leave the other parts relaxed.[1] The snakes are learning to move.

Phase two: With relaxed arms, shoot your hands out into a wedge. Take your hands and shoot them out along the centerline. Hold your elbows like I showed you in the last chapter. Keep your hands and wrists relaxed and raise your arms as if you were flicking water into someone's face. Drop your arms to your sides, and then shoot out again. The snakes are striking.

Phase three: Shoot your arms out again, then lock down your muscles at the end of the movement. It's important not to lock your arm muscles from your hands back. Do it from your back muscles forward up your arms. Your upper arm tightens, but your hands can be relaxed. Once you lock down your muscles, relax again and drop them back. The snakes are constricting and then resting.

Phase four: When you get to a chosen point in the block, tighten up. Notice I didn't say at the end of the block—that was before. Now, anywhere you tense is the end of the block. This is important, and I'll go more into it in a bit.[2]

There are beaucoup important reasons to do these exercises. I could give you a long-winded explanation as to why they're critical for breaking you out of muscle memory patterns, establishing new neural pathways and associative patterns, but I don't want to get yelled at by my editor for going off on an unnecessary tangent. You'll just have to take it on faith that you will learn lots of important stuff doing this.

The positioning of your hands on your centerline gives you a superior defensive position. The relaxed arms give you speed, and tensing them gives you power. On the last point, simply by learning how to separate them you get both speed and power. Not a bad combo, is it?

Don't worry that your attacker will come charging through these soft-arm defenses—that's why you tighten at the end. Wait a bit and I'll tell you something that will definitely cause bad news for him if he tries. It involves his hitting that wedge, and that has all sorts of nifty effects on his vertical axis. When they all come crashing into the guy at once it really rains on his birthday.

With all this weird muscle tension stuff, you are learning to hit with not only speed and power, but your entire body weight. These kinds of blows are devastating and will knock you senseless. There are two ways of doing them—the complicated way and the easy way. I'm showing you the easier, more bulletproof way.[3] I want you to stop and think about the implications of that for a second. If this is the easy way to deliver maximum speed and power and a) you've never heard of it, b) it's got your head spinning, and c) you're going to have to go out and spend a lot of time figuring out how it works, how

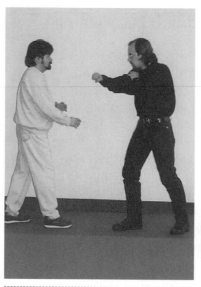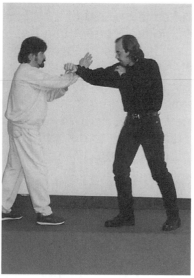

Wedge

likely is it that some punk is going to be able to deliver such an effective blow? To really put it in the "snowball's chances" category, odds are even if he knows about it, he's going to be trying to do it the more complicated way! Meanwhile, you're doing exactly what he can't figure out how to do—hitting with everything you've got!

Let's look again at the photos we saw in the last chapter.

Here is a point I have a really difficult time getting hard stylists past. While it's tempting to block like that with a fist, it is much better to block with an open hand. The reason it's better is you have many more options with an open hand than with a closed fist. An open hand allows you to check, strike, grab, rip, or generally annoy your opponent in all sorts of entertaining ways.

What I also want you to realize is that the real block was done with the wedge. All the extra check,

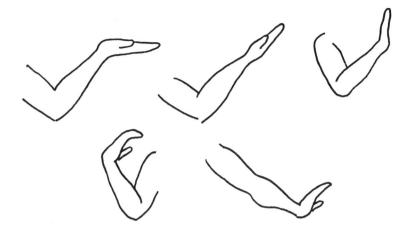

sweep, grab, open, fold, spindle, and mutilate stuff
that follows is pretty much the icing on the cake.
The wedge/triangle has blocked his attack, and the
rest of the stuff you're going to lay on him is
designed to make his life so miserable that he
won't have a chance to attack again.

There are many more ways that I won't go into.
However, notice all the different ways that your
hand can end up. Within the small motions of hand
positioning are very, very important issues of
physics, torque, spin, pop, and other rude surprises.
These lurk just under the surface, like a shark looking for lunch.

Something that will help you to effectively
apply these is an exercise I call "draw the
bow/spin the wheel."

It's another one of those "why it works would
take too long to explain" things, but work it does.
First, stand up and extend your hands in front of
you. Pretend you have watches on both wrists and
look at them at the same time. Then lock your arms
down the way I told you—from the back out. Now
spin along your vertical axis. Go in both directions.

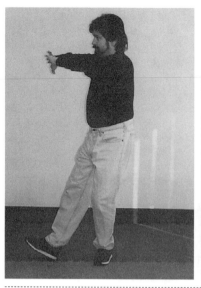
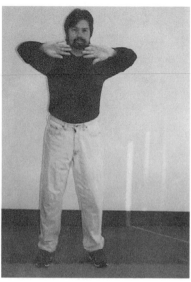

Spin the wheel left/center/right

This is "spin the wheel." You may not realize it, but this action puts your entire body weight behind your hands and arms. You have a nasty push/pull action going on using serious mass instead of muscle. For that added Machiavellian touch, instead of just spinning as you move, bend your knees. This causes you to corkscrew down. Major power is generated in that simple move.

Next comes "draw

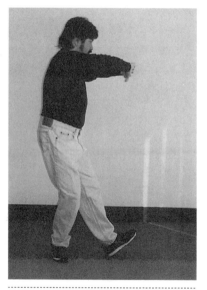

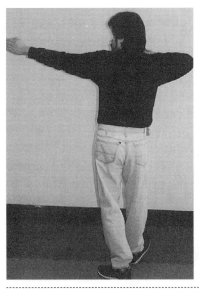
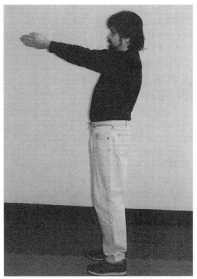

Drawing the bow left/center/right

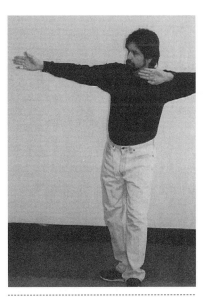

the bow." Extend your hands out, then spin around your vertical axis, keeping one hand out as if it is holding a bow. The other hand comes back as if you are drawing the string. The arms are relaxed and moving. Do it in both directions. Once you can do this, instead of just drawing the string add that extra wrist twist as though you were looking at your

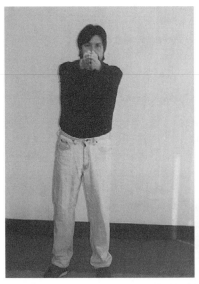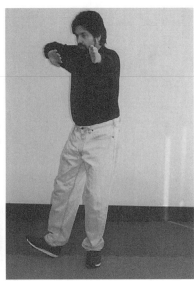

Draw bow/spin wheel

watch. This results in your nose pointing at the back of your hand. Another useful variation is, as you pull back, do that wrist flip again and drop your elbow. This results in your fingers pointing up and your palm out. It's almost as if you were waving to someone.

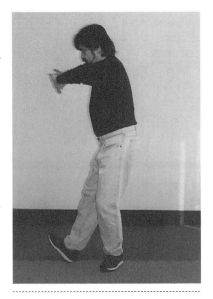

Now combine the two basic moves. Start drawing the bow, but in mid-flight tighten your muscles down and turn it into a spin the wheel. Don't forget to corkscrew down and look at your watch.

Now try it the other way, starting with spin the wheel, then turning it into draw the bow. Keep on doing both the individual moves and the combinations until you can flow from one to another as gracefully as a ballet dancer. That's your goal.

While I don't recommend you run right out and sign up for the Ultimate Fighting Championship, you now have the basic action for all sorts of nasty throws, blows, breaks, twists, snaps, crackles, and pops. When you learn to follow up a wedge block with this action, I guarantee your attacker won't be loving life—unless he considers getting thrown head first into a wall a fun thing to do on a Saturday night.

It will take loads of tinkering on your part to understand all the neat things you can do with these moves. It's that principle thing, again. Those two simple moves literally have thousands of manifestations since they are the driving force in a majority of takedowns. But until you apply them in whatever takedown you use, you will have a car body with no engine. You may have the form, but not what powers it. What I have just done is put a very big engine in your car. Now you just have to practice driving it.

Like I said, the basic block is in the wedge. What you would normally call a block now serves a different purpose, and that is to blow the guy's defenses wide open for your counterattack. It is no longer to stop a blow, but to be like a Weed-Whacker and clear away all the brush. And now that the way is clear, all sorts of things are going to be entering laughing boy's life.

By the way, I'm not saying to totally forget the blocks you already know and use only the wedge. In many cases, those kinds of blocks will be the only thing you can get up in time. The object of the exercise is not to get hit, so use whatever you can. It's just that I'm sure you will find that incorporating this deep driving wedge will have all sorts of benefits.

But while we're on the subject, in order to improve all your blocks, you have to be aware that your hard style might have programmed you to wait until a certain point before doing a particular move within a move. More specifically, what I'm talking about is waiting until the end of a block before snapping, clenching, twisting, popping, or whatever it is you do to give it more "Oomph." This is regardless of where you actually meet the incoming blow.

I've seen it with beginners and with experts, that's how ingrained it is. With many styles, no matter where you make contact with the attack, the spin, snap, or lockdown is done at the end of the block. That means instead of this move being used where it would do the most good (like the moment you encounter his attack), it's used as kind of a P.S. with an attitude. Unfortunately, that's kind of late. That's like dessert showing up four hours after you've left the dinner table. It's there, but you've moved on, so all it's doing is sitting there melting.

ANIMAL'S IMPORTANT SAFETY TIP

- Don't wait until the end of the move before you add the torque! The moment your forearm or hand makes contact (or immediately before) is when you start the extra motion!

When you add this torque, instead of hitting the guy's attack with just one force, you're hitting him with two forces at once—your arm's motion in the block and the spin/pop/lockdown or whatever you use to enhance it. This is going to cause him all

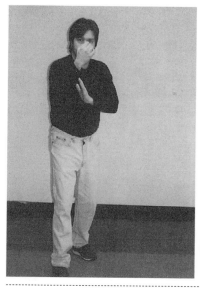
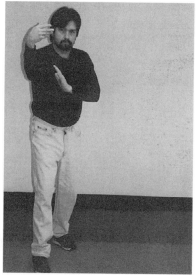

Straight block   Block with side wrist snap

sorts of chaos. If you wait until the completion of
the block before you add that extra twist, you're
losing all sorts of energy that could have been used
to keep him from relocating your nose over next to
your ear.

This is one of the areas where the exercises I just
gave you come into play. But unless you have practiced relaxing, tensing, turning, and twisting at odd
moments, you're not going to be able to do it effectively. While this may sound a little more exact than
you are accustomed to thinking in a fight, realize it's
simply another manifestation of breaking what's
going on into smaller time chunks. It's not just one
automatic motion in two seconds; it's two one-sec-
ond chunks. It's motion/contact, motion/tension.

Let's look at the different open-hand positions.
The first of the open-hand blocks is probably the
least effective, but it will be the one that people
who study "do"-ending styles will be the most com-

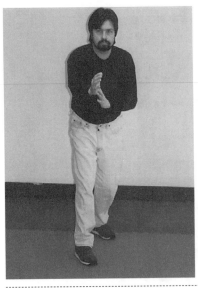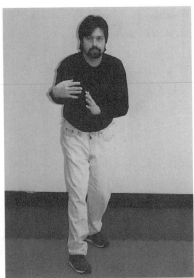

Whip block

fortable with, at least in the transition to open-hand blocks. By adding a small sideways wrist snap, you can make it more effective.

Since I come from styles that place heavy emphasis on subtle hand and wrist movements, I do this instinctively. If you study a hard style it may take you some time to get the hang of it. That's OK. It's a good starting point, and it should integrate nicely with your style.

The next block is a backward whip/slap block that I've explained in mind-numbing detail else-where.[4] From open hands held on the centerline, this is the most direct and shortest block you can do.

Pay close attention to the fact that you can do this horizontally, vertically, and diagonally. That diagonal block can do wonders for keeping your nose from getting rocket-launched through the back of your skull. Add this to that shooting-your-arm-out motion (as though you were flicking water into his

Taking It to the Street

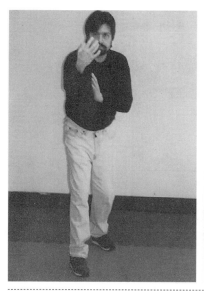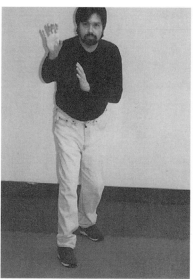

Wrist flip

eyes, remember?) and you get a pretty good combo. No matter how you choose to do this coming off the centerline, this kind of block is faster than a rattlesnake on a meth binge.

I learned the rotating/spinning wrist block from Shaolin five animals and wing chun. You spin your palm around so it's facing your attacker (as though you were looking at your watch). From this position, you can do a plethora of nasty and really effective moves, including maimers (ripping, tearing, and gouging moves),[5] checks (shoving actions against the attacker's arm), or jerks (grabbing and pulling down and/or outward).

Blending that wrist spin with extended arms puts you into a really neat position and him in a really lousy one. It puts you in a perfect position to control his vertical axis. You glom onto his shoulder or upper arm and push and/or pull, and you can mess him up in all sorts of ways. All of these neat

Blocking **149**

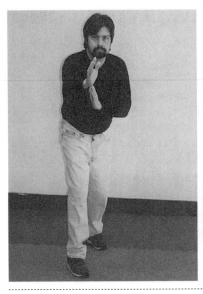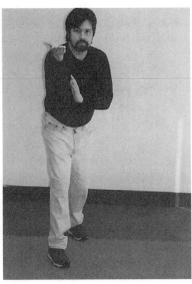

Waiter/kwun sao

things come from simply turning your palm out
toward the guy when you block.

The last block I want you to experiment with has
a variety of names in the styles that use it; however, I
like what Stevan Plinck calls it: "The Waiter Stance."
There are a variety of ways to do this block, and each
has its own name. But what's in a name? A kwun sao
by any other name would still work as sweet.

The proper waiter is when the hand is held flat,
just as though you were holding a tray full of food
(good imagery there). The finishing touch is that
you don't hold your fingers straight forward, but
turned outward toward the diagonal. If your nose is
12 o'clock, then your fingers point toward 2 and 10
o'clock.

While a hand held out either straight out or
skewed works to keep your face from getting splat-
tered, doing that slight twist creates a hook. With
this hook you can snag your opponent's striking limb

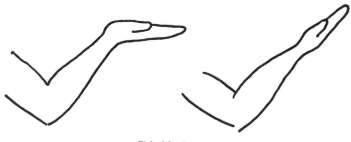

Side block

just long enough to whip around and grab it with your hand. I have to tell you, few fighters are experienced enough to recognize the danger of their limbs being hooked or grabbed. In case you haven't noticed, this is one of the reasons aikido and jujutsu are so effective—by the time the guy recognizes a hold on his arm as a threat, it's too late.

The really fun news is that most people tend to fight the hook instead of trying to escape by outrunning it or slithering out. They often push back, which puts them deeper into it. Their habit of foolishly hanging around like this gives you time to spring the real trap.[6] If all else fails, you can just fire a palm strike into his face from this position.

One of the disadvantages of a flat-handed block is that, while it works great moving to the outside, it's somewhat clumsy crossing

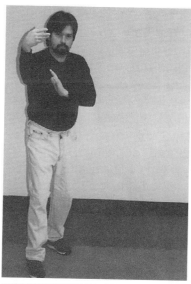

Block with side wrist snap

over your body. If you hold your hand diagonally, it works better on an inside block.

Naturally, this move works better if you pop your wrist in the same direction that you're blocking. This chopping action with the side of your hand and wrist adds energy to the block. So does having your wrist and hand relaxed and flopping your hand over his arm like a dead fish.

From this position, you can whip around, placing your palm on his arm, and check his arm aside or grab him and jerk. While that may not sound like much, wait until we get into the offensive centerline chapter, and you'll see what kind of fun things you can do to someone from this position.

I want to take you back for a second to the beginning of this chapter and the explanation of how tight/loose your arms need to be. Actually, I want to take you back where I said I'd give you the answer to crossing your arms. The answer was in the beginning of this chapter. Crossing your arms is only a problem if you stick them out there all tightened up. If the guy slaps your hand, you end up fighting the blow instead of escaping. In doing so, one tree branch gets knocked into another. You get jammed up, messed up, and crossed up—which is not good.

Think snakes. Your hands writhe around each other like two snakes racing toward a mouse. If someone slaps your lead hand, don't fight it! Let it pull away from the blow. I don't care if he slaps it down, knocks it into your rear hand, or tries to climb over it, let it go. The reason it doesn't matter is your rear hand snakes over the hand being slapped and reclaims the centerline. The other snake gets the mouse. Your slapped lead hand, in the meantime, slips out of the way and recoils to the rear position. It knows there will be another

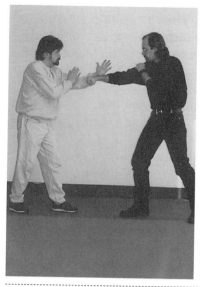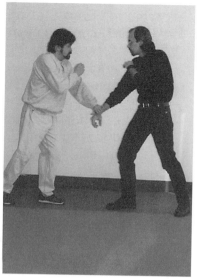

What happens with tight arms

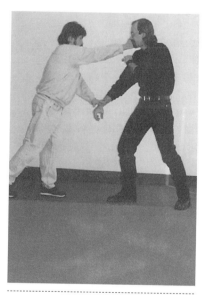

mouse coming along soon.

There is no way I can describe how frustrating it is to fight someone who does this. About the closest situation I can think of is trying to pet a cat that doesn't want to be touched. When you reach down to make contact, the cat just wriggles out of the way. Somehow, they can twist, flatten, and squeeze their bodies into areas where you wouldn't think they'd fit. They shouldn't be able to do that! If you've ever had that same cat suddenly flip around and muckle onto you with claw and fang, you have an idea what it's like to run into that back hand. Now imagine that instead of your hand, it's your face that cat gets ahold of. That is exactly what is going to happen if the guy tries to slap your hand down and charge in.

If your hands and arms are loose, you can do this easily. If they are sticking out there like branches off a tree trunk, you're going to find out why your sensei said don't cross your arms. As I say again and again to hard stylists . . . RELAX!

To get the basic action, pretend you are a choo-choo train. Stick your hands out in front of you and move your hands forward and back as though they were the drive shafts on the wheels of an old steam engine. One pistons up and out, while the other pistons down and back. Once you have that action, turn it into snakes slithering over each other to get the mouse on the end of your attacker's nose.

That's one way of handling that problem. Another way sounds so utterly weird that until you try it you won't believe that it makes such a difference. Basically, you brace your block. I learned this move from silat, and it totally blew me away with its effectiveness. By bracing his or her arms like an A-frame, a person who is smaller, weaker, or older, can prevent someone with greater upper body strength and mass from powering through a block. Neat stuff, Maynard!

I love this braced block. Go out and work with it, especially if you aren't that big and strong or if you are a woman.[7] This braced block allows a smaller person to withstand the wave attack of a larger opponent. By putting your backhand up as a brace and pushing it at the attacking side's hub

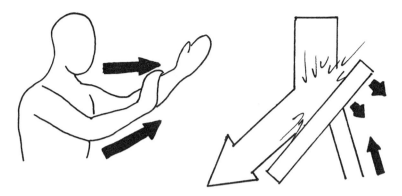

Braced block   Force meeting brace

(forward) you create a structural integrity that far exceeds your muscle strength. Your arms are suddenly the in-the-field representatives of your entire body weight. In order to blow through that structure, the guy you're facing would have to have had several generations of pachyderms in his family tree. And I'm not talking about no tiny Indian elephants, neither.

What he's not going to be able to do is muscle his way through. When you stick your arms out like this, you are putting a concrete divider down your centerline. Like those suckers on the freeway that can bounce a car off without moving, it keeps traffic on either side. And good luck trying to push your way through.

This is more stable if you put forward the same leg as your lead hand. There are all sorts of reasons for this, but we'll go into them later. What I will tell you now is that you achieve a massive shielding effect by either stepping forward or back to match hand and lead.

The backward version is really important if some bozo decides to unexpectedly launch himself at you in a wave-like attack. That back step is not a retreat, just a strategic withdrawal into some really

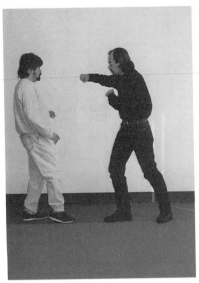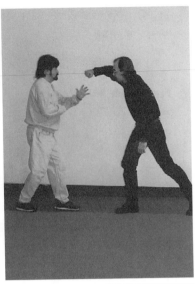

Braced wedge against his entire body weight

bad news for him. His blitzkrieg that seemed to be going fine a second ago is going to unexpectedly ricochet off a solid wedge. The application of this one step back and braced block becomes real clear in a cramped area where you can't go back too far and someone is trying to have your eyeballs as an appetizer.

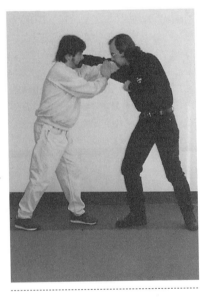

Let me tell you a story about how effective this move is.

A large metro police department sent two officers to check out my professional use of force program for in-service accreditation. As well as being training officers, they were from the gang unit. The lighter one outweighed me by 110 pounds, while the other guy was double my body weight (he was also a power-lifter). We took one look at these guys and immediately dubbed them Godzilla and Ghidra. No lie, these guys were so big that by merely ducking my head, I was able to walk underneath their arms. By using this braced block, I not only kept them from knocking me into next week and prevented them from bowling me over, but I even managed to repeatedly put them down on the ground. And they were not pulling their punches, either. One guy went flying off my block when he threw a blow at me backed by his entire body weight. I had to turn and chase him! If this move works on these monsters, you can be assured it will work on whatever problem you're facing.

Modify this concept to whatever style you study or fighting stance you like. What I would also suggest is that you not only work with it with side stances but learn what it can do from the front. (Not a "front stance," but starting from a normal standing position, stepping backward and throwing your hands up.) Practice both grounding (stopping at one step and digging in) and backpedaling (keeping on moving back) while doing it.

The reason for this is simple: If somebody decides to launch at you, odds are he's going to do it when you're standing normally and *not* in a fighting stance. Whipping your hands up the centerline into a braced block and stepping back will keep him from landing anything solid.

THREE STRIKES, YOU'RE OUT

Let's take a quick trip down memory lane. In my first book I mentioned the three types of blows: Set Ups, Rattlers, and Nighty Nite Bunny Rabbits.[8]

Nighty Nite Bunny Rabbits

Nighty Nite Bunny Rabbits (NNBRs) are massively powerful blows that end the fight when they land. They don't have to be knockouts per se, but they do tend to take the fight out of the guy who catches one. These are things like hanging punches, shin kicks, and that nasty elbow that unexpectedly shows up out of nowhere. They are effective because they put all your body weight into a blow and get it all there at once.

Remember when I said that the moment he is attacking the only thing you have to concern yourself with is that attack? Well, with NNBRs you'd better focus only on defeating that attack; otherwise you're not going to be noticing anything else except pain for a while afterward.

The good news about them, however, is that they are often (relatively speaking) slow. They usually hide behind a few lighter punches that come in first to soften you up. These are often what are called "finishing blows" in sports combinations. They are also pretty rare because they require lots of practice and coordination that far exceeds walking and chewing gum at the same time. The guy may be trying to throw NNBRs, but all he is actually doing is throwing Rattlers.

Whether you're up against a trained fighter who knows how to throw NNBRs or someone who is only the second generation in his family to walk upright, the braced block and moving are your best chance against these and other power attacks. Whether the motion is forward into your attacker (against a shin kick[9]) or backward and out of range (against elbows and ugly punches), the brace should keep you safe.

Oh yeah, when I say move into an attack, many people look at me like I'm crazy. They think I just said run directly toward the car that is going run over them. Not true. A moving car has no optimal point of impact; it's mass in consistent motion. Wherever it hits, it will cause damage.

However, a punch is *not* like a moving car; it's like swinging a baseball bat. There are all sorts of things going on to complicate it (ergo, mess it up, too). A second ago, it wasn't moving; now it is. That means it hasn't picked up speed yet, AND it's moving around a hub—not in a pure straight line. In order for it to be effective, the body mass has to be moved behind it. On top of all of that, there is an optimal point! Before that or after that, it isn't nearly as effective! Sticking with the baseball swing analogy, if you hit it right you get a home run. Miss that point and you get singles, fouls, errors, and pop-ups. That's if you don't strike out all together! I'll go into it more in the next chapter, but for right now keep this idea of getting out of the optimal point of impact in the back of your mind.

Rattlers

The next type of blow is called a Rattler. While some might say that they are so named because they can snake in like a striking rattlesnake, the truth is I call them this because they can rattle your eyeballs in your head. Properly thrown hooks and jabs from a boxer constitute Rattlers. Unlike the NNBR, these suckers do cumulative damage. Take three of these suckers and your brains are going to be shivering and shaking worse than a nekkid stripper in a Montana snowstorm.

Fortunately, because most people don't know how to throw an effective punch, odds are that guy coming at you in the wave attack in the locker room is just going to be throwing Rattlers. He may think he's throwing NNBRs, but his inability to do that pedestrian and gum thing is going to keep him from throwing truly devastating blows.[10] Most Rattlers are thrown with only arm muscle behind them; however, they can get varying degrees of body weight behind them. If enough land, you're going to be in trouble. But the odds of a one-punch knockout are rare. This is good news because Rattlers are easy to block.

Want to know the amazing secret behind this mystery blocking technique? Not to disappoint you, but you know it already. It consists of relaxed muscles, watching the hub, and shooting your hands out along the centerline in a wedge. Once you make contact, tighten up for a second to stop the force, then relax and brush it away while bringing your rear hand forward.

Rattlers can be fast. Add to that the chance that he may have gotten the jump on you throwing the blow. But remember to use the things we've talked about, and you'll beat him to the finish line nine times out of 10. The real trick to this is not to block at the hand, but block as deeply as you can. Reach for the hub. Remember that the circumference moves faster than the hub. Unless you're really quick, you won't get to the hand in time, but you can do all sorts of stuff on the inside of the guy's elbow, on his upper arm, and on his shoulder.[11]

Set Ups
Set Ups are those light hits, fast feints, or sucker attacks designed to make you open up to the real attack. They don't even pretend to have body

weight behind them. If the guy throwing them is any good, they don't have tight muscles powering them, either. That is why they are so fast—the arms are relaxed. But speed is all they have.

These feints are purely psychological. If I want to attack high, I kick low to get you chasing will-o'-the-wisps, and then I charge in with my real attack. If I want you to tighten up and slow down, I snake in a few of these and get you all hairless—then I exploit the reduction of your speed.

To tell you the truth, you won't encounter many of these in real fights. Face it, the guy is coming at you in a wave attack, and subtlety tends to be lacking under such circumstances. Remember, he doesn't want to spar with you—he wants to hurt you NOW! He may fake with a kick to the groin, but most often these are clumsy attempts that are easily recognized as such. (Free hint: If the supposed attack suddenly begins to go back to where it started, odds are it was a fake, so stop chasing it and look for the real attack coming in.)

You will find these in sparring matches and tournaments. As a matter of fact, in those circumstances, they are thicker'n fleas. They are fast, non-damaging blows that rack up points. The back fist is a prime example. It's lightning quick, snakes in from unexpected directions, and is great for scoring. It also gets people real cautious about getting close to you. But it would never be able to generate enough power to cause serious damage.[12]

While I don't claim to be a sports fighter, I will tell you that keeping your centerline position will help you in your next sparring match against these kinds of moves. So the guy throws a will-o'-the-wisp blow, and you leave to go chase it for a second. Oh, rude surprise for him, your rear hand is there waiting for his real attack. Of course, if he doesn't have something else lined up, you can offer him your suggestion as to what happens next with that rear hand.

I know a lot of this stuff sounds general to the point of uselessness, so let me again stress that you won't know what you're up against in an actual fight until the exact moment. Therefore, training for exact situations is pointless. Only by understanding the principles of what you're doing can you tailor your moves to meet the exact situation. From the general, you can create the specific.

Let me give you an example of how this kind of thinking works. What you are learning to do here is think like a fireman. A fireman never fights the same fire twice. Each one is radically different. Going into a burning building, he never knows exactly what he's going to encounter. He knows about flashovers, backdrafts, and countless other things that could kill him. Every time he encounters one of these, he has a generalized response that he tailors to the specific situation. That is how he survives running into burning buildings. He isn't nuts; he knows how to think on his feet.

That is what you have to learn. And the fastest and best way to do that is to take these principles and play with them in a safe environment. Go out and try this stuff in sparring matches. Then, if you play the circuit, try them out in tournaments. Discover where they work and where they don't work. Try doing them in different ways and see the results. The more you figure them out for yourself, the more effective you will be in both the ring and real life.

---

[1] You may want to work your way up to doing this with your whole body. Then work on doing different parts, like legs, chest, neck, and abdomen. It's kind of useful to be able to

tighten an area up a moment before the blow lands while keeping everything else soft and loose. You can add mondo power to your blows if you learn this trick.

2 Phase five (and this one is going to be a bear folks): Do your katas totally relaxed. Don't throw muscle tension into the process at any point. Your blocks are relaxed, your kicks are soft, your punches are floating out there. Imagine as though you were in a pool and flowing from move to move. In fact, if you have access to a pool, go do your katas neck deep in water. Don't get frustrated or freaked out, however, if you suddenly find yourself flubbing your katas. I've seen black belts drop the ball doing their style's most basic forms while trying this new way. I had the same reaction when my pa-kua sifu told me to do "monkey snatches peaches" softly and gently. I nearly fell on my face. I couldn't do it!

3 As a point of reference, a knockout karate or boxing blow is the most complicated and difficult punch there is to master. There are so many things going on that have to be "juuuu-ust right" that it's a miracle they ever do work.

4 For example, *Surviving a Street Knife Fight: Realistic Defense Techniques*, a video I did with Richard Dobson.

5 I mentioned maimers in my first book, *Cheap Shots, Ambushes, and Other Lessons*. They're not known very well in most impact styles, but are used extensively in kung fu systems. There is a very good reason that I advocate running fiercely from someone who uses them, as they have a nasty habit of tearing off body parts and handing them back to you.

6 This should also serve as good reason for you to train yourself to react immediately to someone's grabbing your arm and wrist. It is an attack. Focus a counterattack on the hand at the same time you break free.

7 Especially pay attention to this idea if you teach self-defense to women and young males. While you may be able to stop a charging 6-foot-4-inch football player's wave attack, those people won't. Don't teach for what you can do, teach for what your students can do.

Blocking

8   *Cheap Shots, Ambushes, and Other Lessons* and, yes, the name does come from a cartoon. I'll give you a hint as to which one; it's got a smart-aleck rabbit and a big orange monster in it.

9   Back when I wrote *Cheap Shots,* I called them stick kicks. Since then I've heard them called shin kicks, Muay Thai kicks, straight-leg kicks, etc. But no matter what you call them, they are real painful.

10   Of course, your moving from the optimal point of impact can greatly aid in fouling up the process too, ya know.

11   You should know that by striking/blocking at the hands and wrists, you can get more leverage on the guy's arm. There are two problem with this, however. One, you have to be *real* fast, accurate, and sensitive to do this. Two, if you mess up in the slightest way, you're left flapping in the wind. His blow has a really good chance of getting through and nailing you. Going deep is easier, safer, and more reliable in a real situation

12   This is in large part due to the structure of the elbow. Because of the way it bends, it cannot brace itself enough to inflict damage. On the other hand, its close cousin, the hammer fist, causes a bone rotation that allows the elbow to brace. It can give you a headache.

CHAPTER 8

Offensive Centerline

....

The philosophy of this style is, 'I hit you.'
Not much on sophistication are you?
It works.
Good point.
    —A conversation with my silat instructor

One of the things I have noticed in many martial arts is what I call the "fencing attitude." In modern sport fencing, there is a thing called "right of way." This simply means that you trade off attacking or defending. If he launches an attack first, he has right of way, and you must defend. After you have blocked, you have the right to riposte (take a poke at him), and then he must defend. In light of the fact that you're playing with representations of giant straight razors, this idea of attack/defend makes sense. The thing about right of way is it leads to a timing of "bomp de bomp de bomp de bomp." Attack, defend, attack, defend, etc., until someone skewers his opponent.

During martial arts sparring, it is the same thing—they block, they attack, they block, they attack again "bomp de bomp de bomp." Well, OK, so it more often goes: attack (flail wildly), WHAM! "Break, point!" You see what I mean, though.

Let us look to the wisdom of St. Frank Zappa, who in the song "Dancing Fool" said, "Got no natural rhythm/but when they see me coming, they just step aside." With these sage words, we shall prove once and for all that having no rhythm is not a bad thing. See, my idea of rhythm consists of "bomp WHOMP!" The rest is silence because the fight is over.

Nowhere is it written that you can't do two things at once. You can walk and chew gum at the same time. You can listen to the radio and do your homework. You can defend AND attack at the same time. In boxing it's called counterpunching. In real life, it's called "a jolly good idea" (well, it's called that if you're in England. Use your own local version if you're in Podunk, Iowa).

Counterpunchers are a bear to deal with. They are walking, object lessons as to why you need to keep your guard up while attacking—which most people don't do. Well, guess what? With what you're going to learn in this chapter, you are going to be able to counterpunch and a whole lot more. With this knowledge, you can really mess up some aggressive jerk's plans of dancing on your face.

Go back to the idea of 2-year-old kung fu. To whom does the centerline belong? ME! And what is mine is mine, and what is yours is mine. Just because my lead hand moved from the centerline to block an attack, does that mean I'm giving up my centerline? Uh-unh. It's still mine. That rear hand will be coming out and proving it, too. The second one hand goes wide, the other comes forward. This is what I am talking about when I say shoot your hands forward.

While one hand is blocking, the other is attacking!

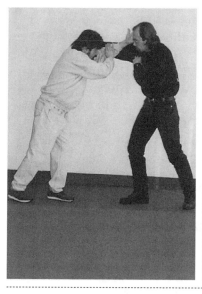

Block

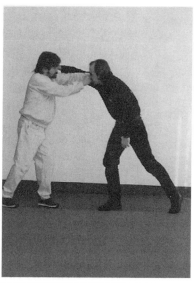

Check body weight

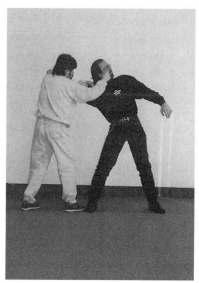

Hit

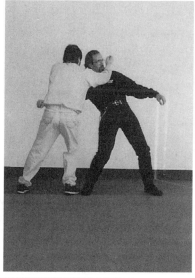

Throw

Offensive Centerline 167

The centerline and everything on it is MINE! MINE! ALL MINE! At all times in all places. That includes his vertical axis. Want to guess what is going to happen when that occurs? It means you're blocking and attacking at the same time.

The 2-year-old attitude has just rolled everything into one. By hogging the centerline, you've just done a bomp-WHOMP! You have combined defense and attack into one ugly move.

The secret of this concept is based on one simple move—stepping forward!

This concept is usually met with the quiet inquiry of "charge into an attacker? Are you out of your mind?" But there is method to my madness.

SIX REASONS STEPPING FORWARD IS INCREDIBLY EFFECTIVE

1) It lessens your chance of getting hit

With the wedge out in front of you, your odds of getting hit are really slim. Add to this that instead of going head to head with him like you're a couple of horny buffalo, you're going to knock him to the side as though he tried to head butt an oncoming snowplow. His attack will be deflected or will just flat out miss. Unfortunately for him, he won't have the luxury of time to stop, reorient, and try again.

2) You're going to crawl right over him

You're not there to fight him, but to go Fluffy the Cat on him. From the moment you say "meow," his major concern won't be winning or what he's going to do to you. It's going to be minimizing the damage as you claw your way up and over him. As you're catting your way out of there, you're going to be hitting him along both his horizontal and vertical axes. When you're crawling over him, which way are you pushing him? Back and down! Your feet and knees hit him in all sorts of tender spots and inconvenient places— many necessary for him to stay upright. He's going to be meeting Mr. Gravity real soon. Go reconsider the horizontal axis chapter in this light, and see how it works in this situation. When you run over someone, you tend to affect him in this manner.

3) You'll control his hub

Do you remember where you aim your blocks? At his hub! You want to get a better hold of it? Move forward. There's something else: That hub is also the outer rim of his vertical axis. Get ahold of it, then snowplow into the guy, and you can really move him. When someone is going one way, it's a real shock when the next thing he knows, he's heading another.

4) His balance is vulnerable

When most people attack, they are not in balance. This is pretty much true across the board. The only thing that varies is the degree. They are expecting to slam into a stationary object (you) over there. They're ready for that. They are not expecting you to jump up, come running across the room, and slam into them! What happens when you get slammed into unexpectedly? Either you fall down or you spend a few frantic seconds trying to get your balance back. That's what slamming into him with the wedge does! He's got to decide whether to keep attacking or do something about sucking earth. Odds are, he's going to opt for the latter. Too bad this is made more complicated by his having to deal simultaneously with the damage you're doing by Fluffying out on him.

If the guy is way out of balance, better known as "overcommitted," the results will be spectacular. A lot of the time, people who punch this way are expecting your face to stop their forward motion. They literally throw themselves at you. Now anybody remember what happens when someone's body weight isn't connected to the ground? What can you do to it much, much easier? Come on, boys and girls, let's not always see the same hands here . . .

That wild, overcommitted blow is going to go severely wrong when it hits the wedge. His body weight is in free-fall, which means it's real easy to affect. All that energy is going to go ricocheting off into the wild blue yonder—usually spinning out of control. Since he is not grounded, this wedge really torques him along his vertical axis.

If that wedge is moving forward at the same time, the disaster is going to be all that much more spectacular. I have quite literally seen attackers throw themselves 5 feet when an overcommitted blow is blocked this way.

5) You'll be out of range

His blow is rigged for delivering maximum force at a particular spot. So, GET OUT OF THAT SPOT! Even if you do get hit by stepping out of the intended range of the blow, you're reducing its power. You've just dropped an NNBR to a Rattler and a Rattler to a Set Up. This is usually considered a good thing.

6) He'll be confused

When your attacker throws that punch, he's expecting one of two reactions: a) it connects and hurts you or b) it sort of connects, i.e., you block or move in such a way that lessens the blow's effectiveness. What he is not expecting is for everything to suddenly blow up in his face. His sole focus is what he's going to do to you. He was expecting you would stay right there and be hit or defend—not

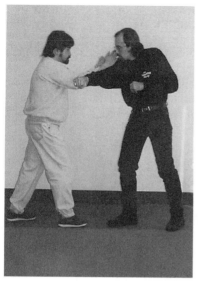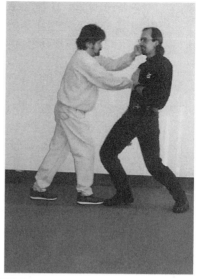

Block   Clear/punch

that he would go whizzing off into space! When those plans go sideways, it is a serious mind bender. And believe me, it's going to take him a few seconds to adjust to the new reality and come up with a plan.[1]

Those six reasons combine to have your attacker going "WHAZZA?" Not only have his plans gone seriously awry, he's disoriented, and he's getting hurt in the process! How would you function under those circumstances? He's not going to be doing so hot either. See, all of a sudden, that stepping forward idea doesn't sound so silly after all does it? Remember Murphy's Law of Combat No. 2? "If it's stupid and it works, it isn't stupid!"

All of these neat things come about because you're being aggressive about keeping the centerline! People trained well enough to handle this sort of attack are few and far between. That leaves a lot of people out there who are big-time suckered by it.

Offensive Centerline   **171**

An untrained fighter or someone with experience in hard styles may even try to throw another punch as you're crawling over him, instead of trying to roll out.[2] Stupid idea, but he may try. So what? It won't have any power. I mean, how much body weight can you get into a blow when you're falling over backward? On top of that, the odds are such a blow will be blocked by your other arm. It's out there too, remember? Besides, stopping damage you'll be doing to him is about to become paramount. All because you chose to step forward instead of standing there and getting punched.

If you study a style in which the fighting stance leaves the centerline open, you've just found a great way to punch a great many of your classmates. Drive the wedge into the hole and start hitting. When they get panicky and try to cover their centerlines, plow into their defenses with a braced wedge from the outside and continue hitting. Subtle no, effective yes.

OK, until now we've been focusing on messing up his centerline as opposed to the vertical axis. Not no more. Here is where the real fun starts. Remember that I just told you most people aren't in balance when they attack? When people are not grounded, unexpected force can play havoc with them. Well, if they spin around the horizontal axis, they also spin around the vertical axis.

In his video, *Practical Hand-to-Hand Combat for the Patrol Officer*, Chris Caracci points out that human beings are oriented on the 90s of their circle.[3] That is to say if you take the person and have him stand in the middle of the Swiss flag, you see how he thinks and orients himself. His nose is zero, his right shoulder is 90, directly behind is 180, his left shoulder is 270. Then back to front. Everything is straight front, straight back, or straight to the sides.

If you watch people, you will begin to see this principle in action. People will look at something and then turn directly toward it. In doing so, they physically orient on it. It's kind of like they get a better radar lock on something if it is on the any of the 90s, especially the line in front.

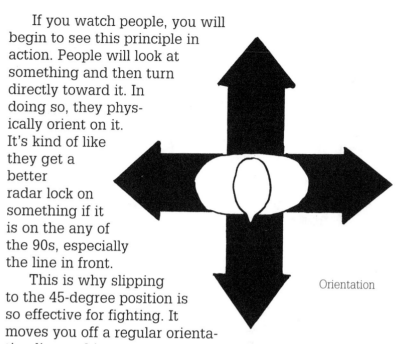

Orientation

This is why slipping to the 45-degree position is so effective for fighting. It moves you off a regular orientation line and into a semi-blind spot. When you move off any of these lines, 99 times out of 100 the guy will stop, do a radar search, pull back to physically reorient back onto his forward line, and then come at you again. Depending on how drunk the guy is, this process can take up to five seconds. If the guy is not bombed, it can buy you at least one second, maybe two.

The really neat thing is that just because you stepped to the 45 doesn't mean you gave up your centerline. It still comes out straight from your nose. As you step, keep looking at him. Your body will adjust itself as you go. You will still have your centerline—just from a different direction. You still have a clear shot to his vertical axis. In fact, it's a clearer shot now that his arms aren't in the way.

By stepping off angle like this, not only do you avoid all sorts of nasty blows and disorient him, but

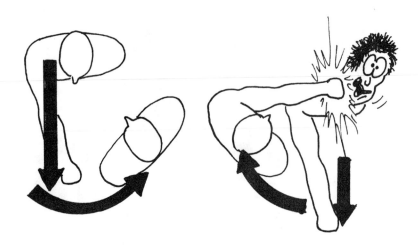

Slipping to 45 degrees and hitting at the same time

you put yourself in a great position to spin him along his vertical axis when you bolt past him. Oh, yeah, you also make it harder for him to catch you, since you are now located on his outside gate, and he has to reach across himself to grab ahold of you. Good luck, sucker.

Hmmm, just a paranoid thought here. For those of you from styles that don't use these terms, inside and outside gates are the two positions you can have in relation to an attacker.

Inside gate means that you are between his arms. The problem with this position is that you are really susceptible to more attacks. From inside gate, you basically have only four options: You can roll the guy back over his horizontal axis by going forward; reach in deep and spin him away from you using his vertical axis (again, forward motion is required); combine the first two; or backpedal. If you backpedal, try to take him over his horizontal axis like I did in the set of photos on page 167. If you can't, try to get out of there in such a way that gets you off his line of orien-

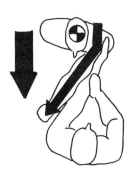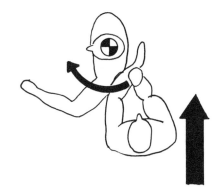

Triangle spin

tation. The option of standing there and trading blows with him should not even be considered.

Outside gate is what we in the biz call a buffet! We are talking a free all-you-can-eat-gourmet-four-star-restaurant-feeding-frenzy here. You can do almost anything from outside his arms. This is a place where the only limit is your imagination. It should be clear by now that it is the position you want to take when attacked.

That's what happens if you move off angle. Wanna guess what happens if you move him off angle? What if you use his vertical axis and spin him around to another direction? Do the words "Application Error" mean anything to you? It's going to mean a whole lot when he spins off like a Frisbee bouncing off a dog's nose.

Most people slam into someone like a square block. In doing this, they don't leave any place for the guy's energy to go except back. While this may sound like a great idea, that ain't going to happen if he's in the middle of charging you. What will result is that you slam into each other and end up doing the buffalo grunt.

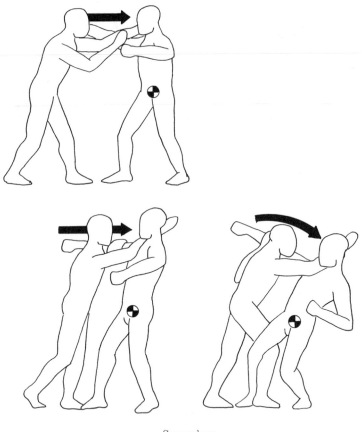

Snowplow

However, if you slam into him as a wedge, you aren't hitting him with a wall. It's a point backed up by two angles that slice through and shed oncoming force. You're giving his energy a place to go. His problem is that he's no longer in control of it. Depending on which side of his centerline you drive into him, he'll spin left or right. Of course, the guy is also spearing himself on the point, which gives him additional motivation to roll off, but that's another story.

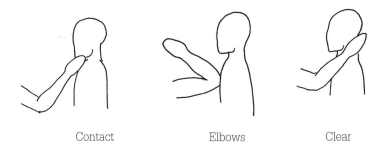

| Contact | Elbows | Clear |

Notice that your hand is hitting near his shoulder, while your elbow is hitting closer to his vertical axis. This combination is important. The further out toward the circumference your hand hits, the more likely you are to get him spinning. (At least until you really get the hang of this idea, then you can zap him from nearly centerline.) Once again let me stress the importance of tightening your muscles from your back, outward along your arms. This allows you to use your body weight, not your muscles, to do the job.

THE IMPORTANCE OF INFIGHTING

The question I imagine most of you are asking now is, "Do I hit with my hand or my elbow?" The answer is, "Yes." Both are valid techniques, and both work. Add your forearm to those two options, and you get all sorts of nifty possibilities. As long as your entire body weight is behind your "shield" (I'll explain that in a bit), it doesn't matter what hits first. Go out and practice all the nifty combinations you can imagine.

Oh, yeah, a point on practicing this stuff; One of the differences between sparring and a real fight is that, in a sparring match, people tend to hang back and poke at each other. This also applies to training; often people hang way back to work on new techniques. While this stuff works under those circumstances, it really comes into its own up close and personal. It is under those circumstances that you need to experiment with this stuff. Have your training partner move in on you when he strikes or be close enough to really hit you.[4]

Colliding with your opponent like a buffalo wanting a hug is one of the things grappling relies on. Enter, break, throw—that's how you do a takedown. Once they close with each other (enter), the person with the wrestling, jujutsu, and judo experience has the distinct advantage. He'll blow your balance (break) and take you down (throw). Then he'll make you regret you were ever born. Most martial artists I know who cross-train tend to train in a distance style (TKD, karate) and grappling. By doing this, they think they've covered all the different ranges. Not so, Grasshopper. They've left out the middle range.

What you are seeing here are examples of infighting. Even though it's close, it's not grappling. It not only messes up the amateur buffalo charge, but it can put a serious dent in the hat of a grappler when he tries to get huggy with you. By using the wedge and elbows, you keep a grappler from getting control of your center of balance or your axes.

As I said before, most people consider infighting to be a transitional range. That is, the neighborhood they have to pass through to get from distance to grappling range. Add to this that I've heard hot debate about whether or not you can stop a determined grappler from taking you down.

Generally, the people having this argument are the same ones who think of this range as transitional. If you know only distance styles and grappling, odds are you can't stop a determined grappler. In fact, any yo-yo charging you has a really good chance of taking you down, whether he's trained or not. But let me tell you, an elbow backed up by your body weight in the face of a would-be tackler can make all the difference in the world.

That is why knowing how to infight is so important. There are a lot of people who can punch real hard from up close, but few can defend from that close. Defending is not just the "cover up and let him pound on you while you play rope-a-dope" of boxing. It means either redirecting his entire body weight or stopping it from slamming into you. It's keeping him out at the length of your upper arm. This keeps him from getting a direct hold of your axes, your center of balance, and your body weight. All of which keeps you from hitting the dirt with the S.O.B.

Whether he's coming at you or you're going at him, it doesn't matter; the principle is the same. However, if you slam into him, you're going to have all sorts of neat results. After impact, spin the wheel or draw the bow. And always push or pull in whatever direction you want him to go and DOWN! Point to where you want him to go.

USING YOUR ELBOWS

Your next gigglefest centers on your elbows. While I can stiff-arm a guy who's trying to rush me, odds are it will slip up and off his chest or face. However, if I plant an elbow into him I do three things: I hurt him severely, I keep him out of grappling range, and I brace myself against his force, lessening my chances of falling down.

I can do all of this by merely collapsing my lead hand against his charge. That lead hand acts as a giant airbag, until he spears himself on my elbow.

If you've ever had an elbow driven into your ribs

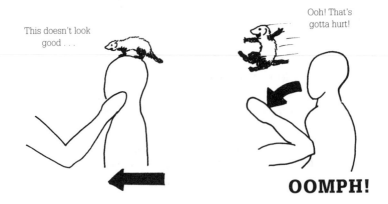

This doesn't look good . . .

Ooh! That's gotta hurt!

OOMPH!

Collapsing arm/impact

(or face), you know how much this hurts. If you haven't, take my word for it, it sucks.

A quick reiteration on muscle tension. You don't stick your arm out and "make a muscle." The way most people do that (and the way they do their karate blocks) is they clench their fist and forearm. If you have a friend around have him push against your fist with his body weight and see what happens. Unless your friend is built like Ichabod Crane, your arm will slowly collapse in.

Instead of trying to make Arnie jealous of your bulging biceps, do it backward like I told you. Tense your muscles from your back and down your arm. Now have your friend try to push his way through that sucker.

This is the difference between an egg and a sumo wrestler. An egg is hard on the outside, but soft and gooey on the inside. Once you're past the hard part, it's easy sailing. A sumo wrestler may be soft outside, but underneath he's pure muscle. It's when you've gotten past the soft part that you realize you are in deep, deep trouble. The closer you get, the harder it gets. Unfortunately, most martial artists are more eggy than sumoish.

This muscle tension pattern is what I call "the shield." These are exactly the muscles you use when you hold a shield and are trying to keep your head from being split open by some psycho with a broadsword. (Don't ask how I know this.) Imagine you have a shield on your forearm and are moving it around. If you hold your upper arm muscles tight like this, not only have you created a buffer up close, but you can keep your forearms relaxed and quick for all those neat blocks I showed you (and all the neat grabs I will show you).

This muscle tension creates a direct line to your body mass and guarantees to make his charge very unpleasant. Instead of running into a square block, he's now running into a spear with its butt firmly planted in the ground. Can you say "ouch," boys and girls? I knew you could.

Notice the three positions the elbow can take. I've rated them on their effectiveness in stopping someone's body mass. Realize that the guy's force is going to be slamming into you (or yours into him). Even with your arm tensed, there's still a chance that it might collapse if you're not in the right position (or braced). The first position is OK. It will work, but there is a chance of its collapsing against his body weight. While this position is great for blocking punches and kicks with your elbows (didn't think about that one did you? Hee, hee, hee—sneaky thing this triangle, isn't it?), it can still potentially fold on you.

The answer to this problem is simple: Twist your body slightly so the elbow is pointing directly into the incoming force.

While this brings the guy a little closer than you

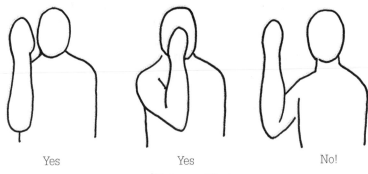

Yes Yes No!

Elbow positions

might like (i.e., almost into grappling range), the motion that puts your elbow into position also can be used to get the chump off you. If you add a shove/strike with the other hand (look at your watch), you're going to really tweak the guy's vertical axis. The combination of slamming into your elbow, getting clobbered, and being knocked aside all at once is going to really ruin his day.

Oh no, not another quick aside! Yep, sad to say, but true. This kind of impact is exactly the same kind you use to break a board. You hit through him. Not only do you impact on him, but you keep driving him down and away. While I ordinarily recommend ending your blow in the middle of the target, in this case push through. You DO want to move him. By punching through him, you end up shoving him. When you run out of arm, just walk forward and reload.

Here's the really fun part. With a little practice you can get to the point where you direct the way the guy flies. If you are up against multiple opponents, instead of throwing him down, you can throw an attacker into his friends. It's great fun to watch them go tumbling down together.

Anyway, back to the issue at hand. (Stay on task, Animal! What can I say? ADD.) The second way to

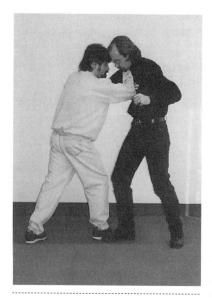

hold your elbow against an impact is straight out. This creates a direct line between your elbow and your body mass. Any force striking it will be hitting head-on, like that braced spear. Guess what? If you plant this into somebody, odds are it won't be directly onto centerline. That means the sucker is going to spin. It's a mini wedge in and of itself. For those of you who didn't notice, that elbow position is exactly the same one you'll be in when you block from your side of centerline. Nifty how this all fits together isn't it?

The third way of holding your elbow is a disaster waiting to happen. By holding your elbow out to the side, you lose the structural integrity of this move. Even if you can do "flies from hell" on the weight machine, you just won't be able to keep your elbow in place to effectively handle his body mass slamming into you. It will peel your defenses open like a grape, so keep the elbow either in front of you or in.

For those who haven't caught on, simply position your elbow in one of the first two positions and step forward. You've just skewered the sucker like a shish kebab. You drop a shielded elbow powered by a drop step into someone, and the guy is going to know it.

WHAT NOW?

Since this is the offensive chapter, let's look at what you do after planting an elbow in the guy as you run over him. Want to know one of the biggest secrets for winning a fight? Here it is: If you've done something that works, don't fight it! IF IT'S WORKING, DON'T FIX IT!

I have seen countless martial artists do something really effective to put the guy down and then stop the guy's fall and drag him back into the fight! The one that gets me really hairless is when they deflect a knife strike and then drag it back across their body! No lie! What they are doing is reacting to their training, not what is happening!

Aikido is really, really bad for this. If the guy is falling, aikidoists will often grab him and drag him back up and toss him in another direction. This often blows up in their faces. In their defense I have to say, the idea behind it is a good one—if you're fighting a trained hard stylist. Such a person will often start to resist the throw. In doing so, he sets himself up for the change in direction by the aikidoist. The next thing he knows, his counter has just been countered!

HOWEVER, many aikidoists mess up by doing the move automatically, just like they practiced. They don't pay attention to what is happening. They get the guy going down, and if they had let him go, he would have fallen. Boom! End of conver-

Best elbow position   Bad elbow position

sation. But instead of letting him fall, their supposed counter *rescues* him! Since the guy isn't resisting, that change in direction doesn't disorient him. It gives him a moment to realize that all hell is breaking loose. Want to guess what his natural reaction is going to be? He's going to grab ahold of the aikidoist like a crawdad and hang on for dear life. Guess who all of a sudden has someone's body weight dangling off the end of his arm? It's supposed to be the other way around, Bozo.

This is what can (and does) happen if you just do moves by rote. Once you got the guy going down, LET HIM GO! In fact, speed him on his way! That's why the elbow check and shove are so effective—the guy bounces off the elbow and then gets sent speeding along the way he just bounced! You're not moving his mass from a stationary position, you're slamming into him in the same direction he's already moving—which makes it real hard for him to control or recover from that fall!

Let's look at the application of this concept. Say after he slams into your elbow, he spins to the outside. There are two ways to handle this. One is the shove I already mentioned. The other is to simply straighten out your arm again and sweep him aside as you go thunderin' past him.

Again, the trick isn't to just move him to the side, but to also move him *down*. Remember, you end up pointing to where you want him to go (i.e., the floor). This is an application of the old "hard to resist two forces at once" issue mixed in with a strong hint of Fluffy. So when you're moving forward and climbing over the guy, this move will be a natural reaction.

Notice how your hand snakes into the juncture of his neck and shoulder after the strike? That is a really secure and easy hold, but not the most dam-

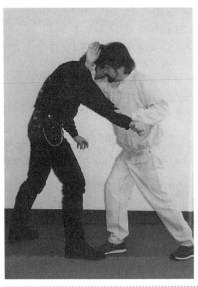
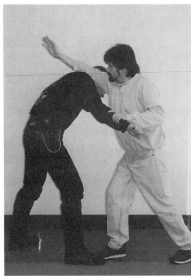

Elbow/sweep

aging. Silat, kuntao, and aikido players will do this same motion by slapping a hand on the guy's face, whipping his head around, and doing a downward pull. While this is devastating, it takes lots of practice. It also can do serious injury to your opponent. This may sound peachy keeno right now, but you'll change your mind when he sues you. Or you may hurt a friend worse than you

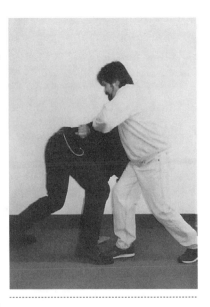

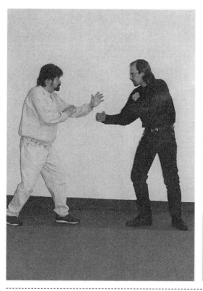
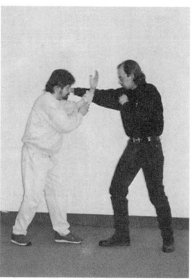

Wedge with the same-side crane

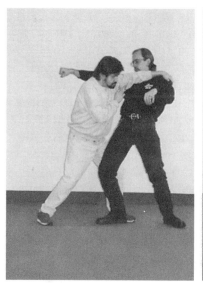
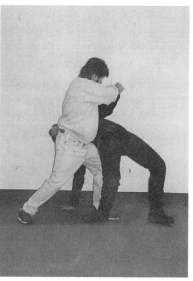

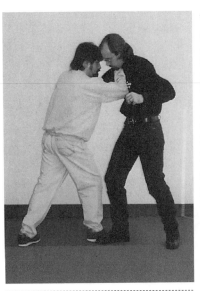
See the hit now?

wanted to. So stick with the safer and easier hold until you get the hang of it. Besides, the sweep looks innocent until you imagine a wall in the guy's flight path. Don't let the fact that I'm talking about escaping fool you into thinking that you can't stick all sorts of horns and sharp edges on this stuff. That's where that mystery hit in Illustration 13 suddenly showed up.

Just by sticking on centerline, you've pretty much guaranteed that you're going to be there to hit him like this as he comes charging in, so use it.[5] The shove works in the same manner, except it's your rear hand that is speeding him along his way. Once he's speared himself on your elbow, your rear hand shoots forward. Instead of draping your lead hand over his shoulder and pulling, you shove his far shoulder around the circumference of his circle. Once you get him moving, the lead hand takes over again, having snaked onto the shoulder/neck junction (which fell into perfect range when you slammed him with the wedge). Once you have a hold, sweep. Pull backward and down, pointing to where you want him to fall.

If he spins to your inside gate when you spear him on your elbow, all you need to do is clear him away with your rear hand. You can do this by either grabbing onto him and jerking or just shooting your rear hand out to his neck junction and sweeping him out of the way. With both, follow your circle

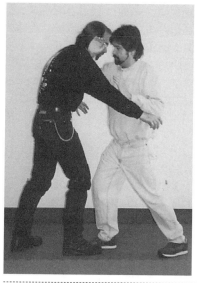

Wedge

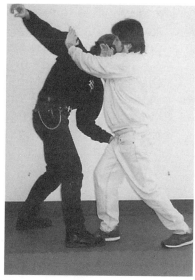

Rear hand shove

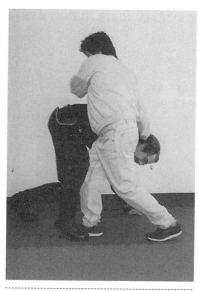

Throw him away

with either a draw the bow or spin the wheel.

While the basic flying wedge is effective in and of itself, if you step on the guy's foot or hook his heel to keep him from stepping back and saving himself as you slam into him, it gets real fun. Go out and experiment with this concept with a friend or sparring partner. Once you understand how it works, then you can add all sorts of bells and whistles to make it nastier. Actually, I should say all sorts of punches, elbows, knees, kicks, gouges, claws, pushes, and pulls.

The very nature of your escape is going to cause the dude all sorts of damage. When you add these extra goodies, you'll often find that in the process of climbing over him to escape, he got so messed up that you "won the fight."

I recently got my first pet ferret. One of Dianna's students looked at me and said, "It fights just like you." Well, yeah. Not only is this little fert totally fearless, attacking things 10 times her size and somehow seeming to attack in 17 places at once, she also has the amazing talent of both running and attacking at the same time.

The reason I bring this up is that I want you to realize a fundamental difference between how a ferret and cat (or a dog) reacts when startled. Most critters will immediately bolt away when grabbed unexpectedly. Then they either keep running or turn and fight back. A ferret, however, even as it's leaping aside, attacks whatever has grabbed ahold of it. What do you expect from a critter that is a first cousin to a wolverine? With that attitude, you can bet that many would-be predators have been rudely surprised when they pounced on a ferret (my cat included—I didn't know he could backpedal that fast).

Adopt the ferret attitude. Get a piece out of whatever is attacking you—even as you wiggle away. If you do that even as you're escaping (if you don't flat out win right then and there), it's going to make chasing you to a place where you are set and ready to rumble a really unappealing idea.

---

[1] This is called "process interruption," and it causes people to go "duh" for a second or two. If you want to see it work in a nonviolent situation, wait until a friend is about to light a cig-

arette and suddenly reach forward and snag it out of his/her mouth. Hold it up in front of them. They will sit there and go "bzzzzt, unable to process data" for a second before they react. Oh, by the way, the normal reaction is usually kind of cranky, so be ready to explain quick.

2   Bailing out of this kind of situation is the easiest way to escape. Literally, you throw yourself into the direction of the spin and get your feet up and out to avoid any trapping. It's called "rolling out." Keep this in mind as you're practicing this stuff with your friends. It will save you lots of bruises. Of course, it would be a whole lot smarter if you did it on mats in the dojo and under supervision instead of on hard concrete or in your backyard. (Hey, I know how these things work.) Like everything else, this is a practiced reaction. It's not something that you are likely to find on your own or do right the first time. But then again, the guy you're laying it on in a parking lot isn't likely to find the right response either.

3   Chris is another one of my "highly recommended" sources for people interested in learning more about application, especially professionally. Not only are his explanations easy to understand, but his video on police room-entry tactics can do wonders for keeping you from getting killed in Doom-like video games. Of course, it also can do wonders for keeping you from getting shot if you really have to search an area for someone with a gun.

4   Oh, by the way, so you don't break your toys, have your partner wear a chest protector whenever you are using elbows. Head gear is also recommended if you are taking him down.

5   Oh, yeah, something that I should tell you—work on your hard jabs, uppercuts, and drop step (all from boxing). All will teach you how to hit very hard in a very short space. Learning how to hurt someone up close tends to make them not want to get snuggly with you. Muay Thai, silat, and kuntao are all elbow intensive, which makes them less than cuddly.

9

Dealing with Kicks

··

*When the opponent attempts to execute a
move, frustrate it from the onset. Make
whatever the opponent was trying to
accomplish of no use.*

—Miyamoto Musashi
The Book of Five Rings

I do have to admit something: I am not a kicker.
My hips are about as flexible as a fundamentalist's
view on sex. This—and a really gruesome experience when a guy launched a front snap kick while I
was in the middle of my spinning heel kick—kind
of closed the book for me on offensive kicking
above the waist. However, that doesn't mean I
don't know about kicking. I know lots about
kicks—namely how to mess 'em up real good. And
gawd, do I love my job!

Most people fear kickers. But when you're done
with this chapter, you're going to do what I do and
hop around chanting, "happy, happy, joy, joy" when
you come across one. That's because you'll know
how to really ruin their day. The trick to all of this is
simplification. Once again, by taking all the different types of kicks and breaking them down to the

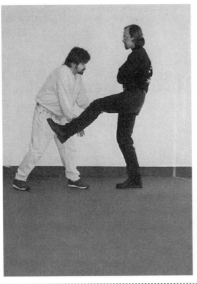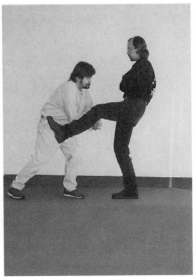

Scooping a kick

simplest components, you find the answer on how to protect yourself from them.

IDENTIFYING KICKS

Here's a real good simplification for starters. Kicks only come in one of two ways—circular or straight. That is to say, with all the thousands of different kicks, there are only two possible ways for them to come at you—straight in or as a circle from the side.

If it comes in straight, the direction is the same regardless of whether he's throwing a front snap kick, thrust kick, side kick, jab kick, etc. This is what the Filipino styles call "an attack on No. 9 angle."

The circle concept is just as simple. A kick is coming in at you along the circumference of his circle. Unless the guy can pull his leg off, the hub of that circle is going to be his hip. From what

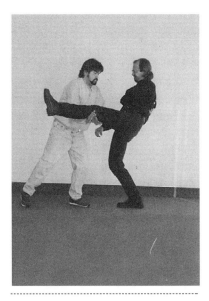

direction will it come? What level will it be on? Or what angle (1-8) will it be on? All of these can be reduced again to our very simple "block left, block right."

Go ahead and play with this idea and see if you can find a kick that doesn't fall into these two categories (good luck). Now if you take this simple concept and mix it up with left/right blocking, the A-frame braced wedge and 2-year-old kung fu, you have a really ugly answer to a kicker. Instead of shooting your hands up and out, you shoot them down and out. If you step forward as you do this, often you can scoop up his kick at the thigh and send him on his head.

ANIMAL'S IMPORTANT SAFETY TIP

- I want to point something out here that is real important to the safety of your training partners. I just told you how to do a motherin' brutal move. Don't do it to your sparring partners! Once you catch his leg and lift it to the point where you know you could take him down, STOP! That means stop moving forward, stop lifting, and, most of all, DON'T shove his leg down into his hips. All of these moves combine

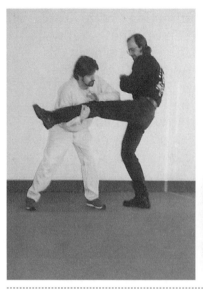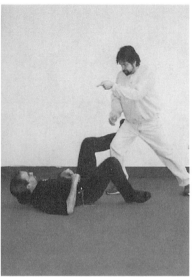

Catch and pivot

into a great way to rip groin muscles and tendons, as well as toss him on his noggin. If you want to learn how to do it, complete the move in your mind, but don't do it against someone you aren't intending to hurt severely.

My normal answer to a kicker is to throw him on his head. However, there will be times that such a move is not what you want to do. A good example of such a time is if he has a friend with him. Under those circumstances, you might want to throw him into his friend, instead.

The way to do that is to simply pivot. That's right, once you have him trapped, simply stick your hand out on the opposite side of the direction you want to throw him and tense your muscles. Now pivot around your vertical axis (follow the circle) in the direction you want him to go.

For the record, this is not a muscle move. It is

the twist from your hips with your entire body weight behind it. The only thing your muscles do once your arm is in place is lock down to deliver the mass of your spinning body.

KINDER, GENTLER KICK AVOIDANCE

I'd like to quickly touch upon a less brutal way to keep from getting kicked. The head honcho at the school I am affiliated with these days has some of the best advice on kicks I've heard, especially for tournaments and sparring matches.

"If a straight kick comes in, get off line. If a circle kick comes in, complete the circle."

That is, if a circle kick is coming at you from the left, step to the right. This puts you on a point farther along the circle. If the kick is coming straight, step either left or right. Well, actually, it's going to be coming in either left or right of the centerline, so figure the shortest route out of there.

EFFECTIVE BLOCKING

OK, remember how I said a blow is designed to deliver maximum impact at a certain point?[1] That is especially true for kicks. Move 6 inches forward, backward, or to the side and the power of that kick has just been seriously diminished. Here's a hint: Odds are that optimal impact point is somewhere really close to where you were standing when the guy started to throw the kick. Within inches of that spot, his kick is going to start losing steam.

This works both ways, into the kick or away from it. You can charge into a kick and destroy its power. But you had better have your ducks in a row before you try it. By this I mean you that have to be damn sure your block is out there before you move.

Dealing with Kicks 197

By shooting your arms out first and stepping in, you destroy the kick's effectiveness and put yourself in a perfect position to scoop and lift.

Until you get to the point where you are effectively blocking this way, I recommend you follow the safer approach of stepping to the side. Aside from the fact that finishing the circle is the safest way to defuse his kick, if the guy is dumb enough to try to hyperextend to get you, he's just handed you his butt on a silver platter.[2]

Oh yeah, here's one more thing about this stepping biz. It applies to both punches and kicks. DO NOT STEP STRAIGHT BACK! The reason is simple. Remember how I told you in Chapter 8 (Offensive Centerline) that human beings are oriented on the 90s? If you step back, you may have avoided a particular blow, but you have done nothing to keep him from continuously attacking! His first attack may have missed, but since you are still in his sights, all he has to do is launch another one.

It's like someone shooting at you and missing. If

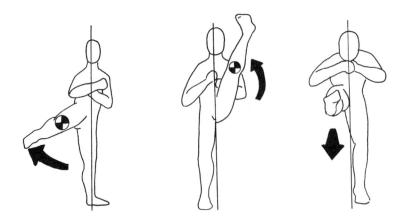

Note knee relative to centerline

Taking It to the Street

you stand there, all he has to do is pull the trigger again and again until he hits you. If you get off line, he has to stop, reorient, aim, and launch another attack. This takes time! While he's reorienting, you can be climbing over him to get out of Dodge.

Believe me when I say I have a lot of experience with backpedaling. Backpedaling may keep you from getting nailed once, but it does nothing to stop the next attack. Getting off line makes him do more work before he

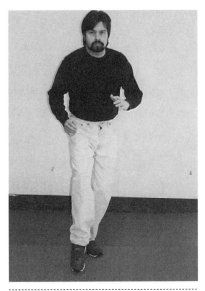

Light foot

can launch another attack. Much more of this will be explained in Chapter 10 (Footwork).

Remember how I told you to figure that the kick is going to come from his light foot? And I also mentioned that the knee is a hub that will tell you where the kick is coming from? It's time to learn how to spot what I'm talking about.

See the centerline? See the hub? His kick will come from the same side of his centerline as the knee of the kicking leg. Take a look at these pictures and you'll begin to see what I'm talking about. Notice how the hub is in the same place for any of the kicks that he throws.

If his knee crosses over the centerline, then he will be coming back with a kick from that new side! Gee, why am I reminded of block left, block right?

I will admit that there is a quasi-neutral ready position for a kick. At this stage, you know a kick

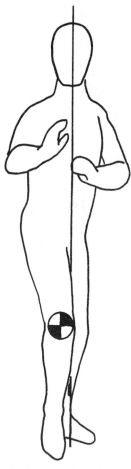

Kicking ready position

is coming, but you're not sure from where.

While in this position, the knee is on one side of the centerline, and he can move in multiple directions. Except for a front snap kick, this position is not yet committed to the actual kick. He's going to kick but hasn't announced where yet. But even with a front snap kick, he's told you it's coming. If that knee doesn't move, it's going to be a straight in kick.

Remember, we're talking about breaking fights down into tiny chunks of time. At this moment, the only thing the guy has done is told you he's about to kick. The exact details may be missing, but he has tipped his hand.

From this position, he is going to have to clearly shift his knee into either of the fields to do a circular kick. If he doesn't do that, gee, think it's going to be a straight kick? This brings us back to the system I just told you about.

I've seen a load of people get real hairless when they see this stance. They don't know what's coming. Personally, when I see this stance, I have a hard time keeping from saying something really tough and macho like "oooh, goody-goody gumdrops." The reason is—unlike most people confronted with this pose—I know what's coming: ME.

If you think a congressman pouncing on a hefty

PAC is fast, you've never seen me move on some fool who does this. The second I see someone do this, my first reaction is "LUNCH MEAT!" especially if he's wagging it out there as a threat.

See, I know something laughing boy doesn't—when he's in that position, he's *reeeeeaally* vulnerable. He's so busy trying to scare me with the threat of a kick, he doesn't realize he has just handed me his balance, his centerline, and about 90 percent of his defensive capabilities. Think maybe I can do something with that?

Laughing boy's agenda is based on your staying right there and getting kicked. And in truth, this is what most inexperienced fighters do. They see that raised knee and hang back going, "Eeek! Freak!" And in doing so, they stay in the guy's effective range! In trying to avoid getting hit, people hang out in the exact place where they will get kicked the most and the hardest! I mean, you might as well just hit yourself. I have to tell you, kickers love it when people get cautious about that dangling knee. It's a natural reaction to back away from things that scare you (unless you're a ferret), but don't stay there—it's bad!

Become that ferret! Attack! You are that 2-year-old! Who does the centerline belong to? Say, "IT'S MINE!" Slam into him with that wedge! You get onto that fool like white on rice! You take that offensive centerline and you ram it down his throat! I cannot begin to tell you all the problems this causes kickers. By going up on one foot, they have sacrificed their base, and, in most cases, their balance. A person on one foot is incredibly easy to spin on either of his axes.

The other thing is, unless he's really well trained, his defenses are going to be weak. Most kickers rely on that offensive foot being the source

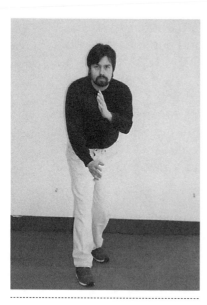
High/low defensive wedge

of their defense. I mean, why bother learning defense when no sane person wants to close with you? Hee, hee, hee, too bad for him, the lunatics have taken over the asylum. I cannot begin to tell you how many people don't guard their groin, knees, or centerline from this position.

Figure when you charge, the guy is going to try to do one of two things. One is he's going to try a thrust kick to keep you back; therefore, expect him to kick. And odds are it will come in straight. But even if he gets slick, a high/low guard as you close will take care of most problems.

If the guy is smarter, he'll try the second option and adjust his distance.

Most people do this by jumping straight back. This is bad for him. Because you have absolutely no reason to stop, you keep on coming in. So while he's bought some distance, he's still on your line of orientation, and you're still going after him, hitting him along his horizontal axis and pushing him down as well as back.

READING THE SIGNS

If all of this sounds incredibly complicated, let me give you an exercise that will help you do it. Like my other exercises, this is a multipart, multilevel training thing. It too starts simple, and yet it is amazing how effective it is when you work your way through it.

Start with a partner standing about 7 to 10 feet away.

He just throws kick after kick. He gets to use whatever kind of kick he wants to—whatever blows up his skirt. But he has to mix and match, that is to say, switch legs, switch kicks. You, in the meantime, stand back and watch. Whenever you see his weight shift over one leg or the other, say "click" or make a short sharp noise. Do this the second you see him shift his weight for a kick. Do this exercise for about 10 minutes or until your partner's legs fall off, whichever comes first.

If you can corral a local black belt into helping you, it's even better because much of his weight shifting will be more subtle and refined. You work at it harder with the black belt, but afterward a junior belt's weight shift will be about as obvious as sunrise.

You'll also begin to see the difference between when a guy is dancing from foot to foot and when he's setting up for a kick. It's a subtle difference, but once you know it, it's an obvious one. It has to do with how high the guy picks his knee up. This also applies to spotting the difference between a step forward and an incoming kick.

The next stage of the exercise is simple. He keeps on kicking and you put your hands out in front of you. Instead of clicking at his weight shift, you point at whichever leg he's kicking with. Both hands point and swing back and forth. As you do this, try to work your way closer and closer to the kick's start. The more you do it, the faster you will become at identifying the attacking leg.

Still keeping your hands in front of you, the third step is to point to whatever direction the kick is

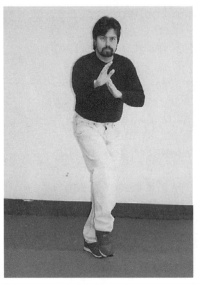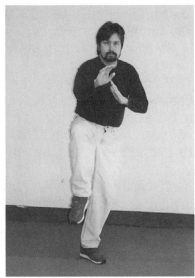

Muay Thai block

coming in from. Point at the kick. If it comes in low,
point low and to the side; if it comes in high, yada,
yada, yada. What is important is that you learn to
recognize the direction a kick is coming at you. You
do this by watching his knee and centerline. Use
either one or both hands to point at the kick (switch
back and forth). This trains you to react left/right
from both sides instead of always blocking right
with your right hand and left with your left.

The final step now that you can see the kicks
coming—still standing seriously apart—is for him to
kick while you step. When he throws a kick you do a
drop step[3] into the position you need to be in to
complete the circle. Do this at first without blocking,
just focusing on stepping away. Once you get pretty
good at this, start throwing in blocks. When you
really get the hang of this, try it in actual sparring.

Do these exercises, and you'll be amazed at how
good you can become at predicting what the guy is

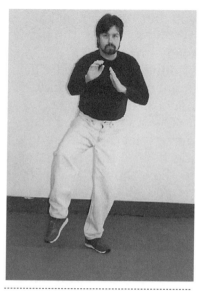

going to throw, kick-wise. Like I said, practice it with black belts who are good at kicking. Once you can predict what's coming from them, kicks from those who are not as advanced will stand out like a brothel in a church district.

BLOCKING WITH YOUR LEGS

Right now I want to show you a really neat trick that works against kicks, knees, hips, and anything else the guy might want to throw at you. While I generally recommend that you get out of the way, sometimes that just isn't possible. So you might as well learn how to block kicks with your legs. While this move works both ways, we'll start inside, moving out.

In a circular motion, lift your knee upward. Do this in such a way that your knee crosses your centerline and your thigh covers your crotch. As it rises up, it crosses your centerline and goes out again. At the top of the circle, your knee should be pointing straight out from your hip. Keep on circling out as you go down.

Do this with both legs from a normal standing position. Then try doing it from your fighting stance. Again, do it with both legs. The first thing you'll probably notice is that it effectively protects your cajones against kicks. I don't know about

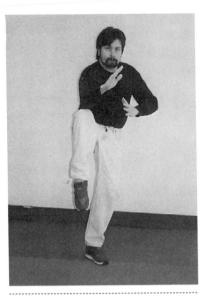
Grasshopper

you, but I always make getting kicked in the nards really low on my list of "things to do today." That is only one of the many benefits of this move.

The trick to doing this move effectively is learning how to rock back and forth as though you were going to kick. Well what can I say? Learning how to shift your weight is kind of critical for any aspect of fighting.

As you get your weight off the blocking leg, whip it upward. Don't hop up onto the supporting leg like I have seen so many people do.[4] The fastest way I know to do this is to just bend the knee of the leg you want to put the weight over. Your lowering one hip allows your body weight to just kind of slip over that leg. In this way gravity, not muscle, moves your body weight. That means you're just a fraction of a second faster, and that counts in this business. Also, the drop tends to pull your kicking leg up for you.

When I asked kickers about that hop, I was told it's supposedly a twofold process that happens in a single, fluid motion (snicker, sure it does). The muscled lift of the kicking leg shifts your body weight onto the other leg and into kicking position. It also powers your leg up and out for a kick. The problem, they said, was that most people don't do those two things simultaneously. Instead, they hop to shift their weight, then shift their body into position for balance, and then kick.

If you want to speed up your leg's getting there, do a move I call the "grasshopper." This move uses your ankle, not your thigh muscles, to lift your leg. As I just mentioned, by slipping your weight onto the leg with the bent knee, you're going to lever your other leg up slightly. Use this slight lift. As your foot is leaving the ground, pop your ankle so your toes point at the ground. This springs you off the ball of your foot. This extra whip combined with your weight shift launches your leg faster and it pops up like a grasshopper.

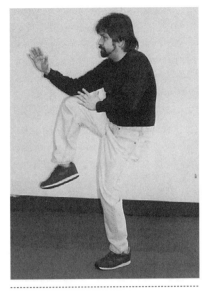

Muay Thai block/shield

Anyway, back to the Muay Thai block. Start doing this move in its exaggerated form of really big circles. Be sure to cross your centerline. Not only does this protect the family jewels, but it sweeps aside straight kicks. What you are doing, in effect, is keeping the centerline with your legs. This is also a really good move against someone who throws a straight kick and then turns it into a roundhouse. That horror-story move doesn't mean squat because you're sweeping out. This blocks both a straight kick AND the roundhouse. Learn to touch your elbow with your knee and you—like a Muay Thai fighter—have effectively shielded your entire side.

Want to know the real fun part of this block? Do it right, and it's offensive. If you have shins of iron, you can turn it out and meet the guy's kick shin to

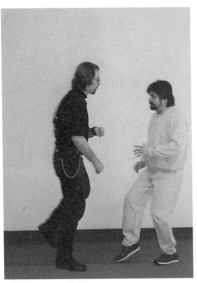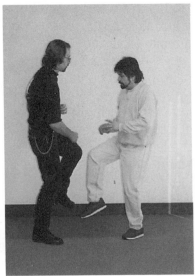

Muay Thai block in action

shin. Believe me when I say few people have shins conditioned to the hardness necessary to withstand this kind of impact. However, being a confirmed wimp, I don't like it because, even if your shins are conditioned, it hurts like a bear. He may not be walking anymore, but you will be limping.

Tell you what, instead of hitting him where he's hard, hit him where he's soft. With a little bit of practice, you can do this block while either lunging or stepping forward and shoving outward with your hips and leg. While it would be loads of laughs to plant a knee in the guy's crotch, unless he's trying to knee you, the odds are that he'll be too far away.

Don't worry, you're going to mess him up in other ways. You can still lunge in and drive your shin into the inside of his thigh. About halfway up on the inside of his thigh is a pressure point (try poking around with your finger until you find it).

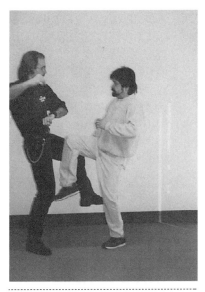

Slamming your shin or knee into this point does three things: It destroys his kick, it hurts like a mother, and it destroys his balance. (Heh, heh, heh . . .)

In the photos at left, I didn't show any sort of hand attack because I want you to focus on the leg work right now. As you can see, though, there are a load of possibilities for slamming him.

ANIMAL'S IMPORTANT SAFETY TIP

- Fighters in general, and kickers in particular, often do not keep a tight defense when they attack! They are so wrapped up in what they are going to do to you that they leave themselves wide open. They are extremely vulnerable to a counterattack. Kickers are the worst; they often leave themselves wide open because they are relying on the distance of their kick to keep them safe. When you counterattack, you not only jam their attack, you come in through the holes they left open.

The outward motion of your leg block's circle is given torque from your hips. Although there is muscle involved, most of the power comes from the hip pivot. Tighten your hips as you block and shove his

Dealing with Kicks   **209**

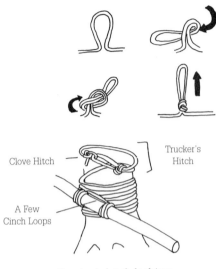

Clove Hitch

Trucker's Hitch

A Few Cinch Loops

Trucker's hitch lashing

kick away. When you get this down, you can spin a kicker like a top. What I recommend is going to a heavy bag (the heavier the better) and practicing slamming it this way. When you get to the point where you can knock an 80-pound bag around like a leaf in a high wind, you'll be able to corkscrew a kicker as though he were a 5-year-old. Remember when I said this motion can be done in either direction? You can do the circle from inside out or from the outside in. Personally, I recommend you get the inside out move perfected before you do the outside in. While the latter is very useful, there are certain situations where, instead of deflecting a kick, it can draw it into your crotch. Not good, this.[5] By knowing how to throw the inside out block really well, you'll know when it's a better move than the outside in.

If you don't have access to a wing chun wooden dummy for this next part, then get a thick pole, some rope (at least 1/4-inch thick), and find a tree. Lash the pole to the tree at a downward angle. Here are some tips on lashing.

No matter how tight you lash it, this sucker is going to come loose, so expect to be tightening it continuously. Do this on a pole instead of a sparring partner because you wouldn't want to hit a friend with the amount of impact you are going to be laying onto this pole.

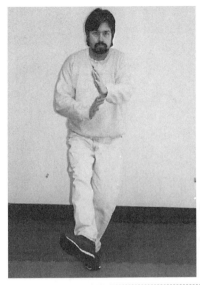 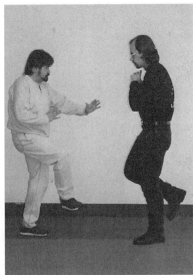

Stomp kick

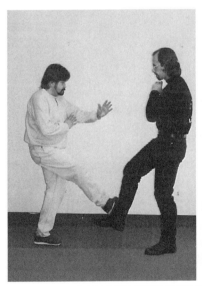 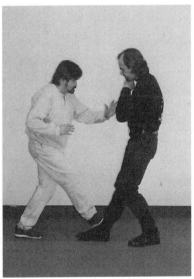

Dealing with Kicks

We're now leaving Muay Thai and moving into wing chun for our kick wreckers. The action is a mix of an exaggerated step, thrust kick, and stomp, all with a little Charlie Chaplin walk thrown in. It feels weird at first, but yee-ha! does it work for messing up kickers! Stand up, lift your knee, turn your foot out to the 45, and kick out at a spot about 2 feet in front of you. As you kick, thrust with your heel.

This is one of the most low-down, nasty, and despicable things you can lay on a kicker. I'm talking, "STBY, Pal." At the very least, you're going to hurt his shin and stop his front kick. At best, you're going to break his foot and knock him over. Most often, you'll get something in between.

So now that you've tied your pole to a tree (BOY! Am I going to let that one slide!), *very lightly* practice lifting your foot and stomping onto the pole. The reason I say lightly is that you will quickly discover why you want to keep the area of impact back toward your ankle and heel.

Before you go for any power or speed, practice accuracy! Otherwise you're going to fold your ankle in half. Get your knee up high and thrust out and down. After you get the hang of it, go into your fighting stance and try turning your lead foot to the inside 45. It doesn't really matter if you do it to the inside or outside 45, but the 45 is important because it gives you a bigger area to block with. This increases your chances of the block working.

This works against kicks that are coming straight in or up from the lower sections. It doesn't really matter if the kick is coming up from a lower angle or is straight in toward your knees or feet. In many styles and tournaments, these are verboten targets, but not in a real fight. In fact, you can tell by someone's fighting stance if he comes from a style where the legs are targets. Styles that allow

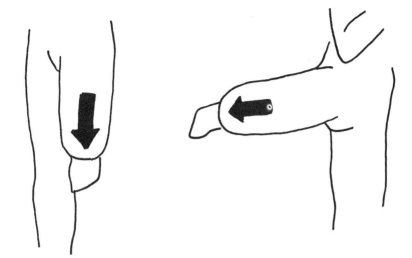

Turn indicator

the legs as targets tend to take more forward-facing stances.

This move is also an attack. You either blow his knee out or you slam it into his shin and rake down. When you encounter ankle, you stomp. Stepping forward to crawl over the guy to escape puts you in the perfect position to lay this on him.

You practice on a pole to improve your accuracy with this kind of block. It's nowhere near as hard as it sounds, especially since I'm going to give you another freebie about kicks. Here it is: Draw an arrow on the guy's thigh above his knee.

It's easy to figure out where a stiff-legged kick is going. Sometimes it's a little harder with a snap kick. His knee is going up one second; the next, ZAP! You get pegged from a totally different direction. That is until you use that arrow. It is going to tell you where his snap kick is going to be. If the arrow is straight up, that's how the kick will be. If it

Dealing with Kicks 213

turns sideways, guess what's coming? The way the knee works sort of forces this to be the case.

By watching this point, you know where his kick is coming from. All you do is put your foot there as if you were working on the pole. Right now, I recommend you work on aiming at the shin (pole) instead of the foot. While such a move can accordion a kicker's toes and foot, it requires an extremely high level of accuracy and lots of practice to get there. The shin, however, will be like a walk in the park.

---

[1] This saying on optimum impact point is another one of Tony J.'s ways of explaining things. If you ever meet him, shake his hand and thank him for this information. You might also want to ask him to teach you to kick. He is good.

[2] Hyperextension occurs when the guy lunges out of his "safety zone" to cover those last 6 inches in order to get you in your new position. In doing so, he overcommits, loses his balance, and locks out his limbs. He effectively "freezes" in that position for a moment. In your "new and improved" timing of fights, it takes him forever to get back to a position where he could keep you from shoving his teeth down his throat. When someone is in this position, you can do all those neat head-thumping techniques you see in martial arts rags.

[3] A drop step is kind of a falling stomp in whatever direction you need to go quickly. I described it in *A Professional's Guide to Ending Violence Quickly*. Jack Dempsey, in his book *Championship Fighting*, was the first person I know who wrote about it. Anyway, it's like walking in that you just collapse a leg and start falling in the direction you want to go. Your hips direct the way you go—just thrust them in that direction. Once you start falling, you shove off with your other leg. To stop, you stomp down with that leg you folded. If you can get a punch to land at the same time as your stomp, it will have your entire body weight behind it. You can easily knock someone into next week doing this kind of move.

[4] When I say "hop" I am referring to this little upward jerk I

have seen many people do. Using the leg they are going to lift up and kick with, they push their body weight onto the other leg. By pushing off in this manner, they do a weird little "hop," which is a dead giveaway that they're about to kick.

[5] I'll give you a freebie, though. Don't use an outside-in kick with your back leg. Keep it as more of a front leg habit.

CHAPTER 10

Footwork

Fighting is like walking through a swamp.
You don't want to stay in one place. You need
to watch where you put your feet, and you
want to get out of there as fast as you can.

—Justin Kocher

I said earlier that you can attack with your feet without ever kicking. This small statement is real important because most people—and I don't care if they're martial artists or bar brawlers—don't protect their legs. In not doing so, they fail to protect their balance, their mobility, and a long list of other things. All in all, this leaves them susceptible to slamming really hard into the earth. Strength, size, and bad attitude don't mean much if you take away someone's balance. The biggest, baddest, strongest dude in the world is not so tough that he's stronger than gravity. Once he meets gravity, he's going down. And all it takes for that to happen is his not getting a foot out there in time.

If you want a warm fuzzy, I have found big guys are very susceptible to this kind of attack. They are so busy relying on bulging muscles that they leave anything below that massive hairy chest flapping in the wind. Take heart. Quite literally, the bigger they are, the harder they fall. And the easier it is to get them to fall.

There are two things that that will help you grasp the importance of this chapter. One you know already: There is a perception that a person resides in his or her head and chest. This is important because it usually means that people leave points south unprotected. You might say it's a target-rich environment down under. The two exceptions to that statement are the pain points, which are to say women's breasts and men's genitals. Both sexes are very cognizant of the potential pain of being struck there, and they do tend to protect those areas.[1] Outside of those pain points, people tend to leave themselves wide open. And that, me buckos, means fiesta time for us!

The other issue I want you to seriously consider is something I have to tell the cops I train—again and again and again. I have said it enough that I have developed a little saying that I continually chant: *"Have faith in a force other than your own muscles!"*

In this little old universe of ours, there are powers greater than your biceps. They were here before your mighty thews came into being, and they will be here long after you have gone away. Once you begin to look into these, brave new worlds will open themselves up to you. It will no longer matter that you are not the biggest, the baddest, the strongest, or the most ferocious.

Having said that, let's look at a few of the forces you can use to make an attacker's life miserable. You will be amazed at the chaos you can cause with just your foot.

ANIMAL'S IMPORTANT SAFETY TIP

- Taking someone's balance away is less a matter of your doing something complicated and more a matter of your simply monkey-wrenching a complicated something that he's doing.

A BALANCING ACT

If you've ever tripped over a crack in the sidewalk, you know how little it takes to affect your balance. Well guess what? Everyone has the same problem. Walking consists of throwing yourself off balance and catching yourself before you fall. The crack you tripped over simply prevented you from getting your foot to where it needed to be in order to regain balance.

Remember when I told you about the missile without the "end task" command in its program? That foot getting out there is the "end task" command. Without it in place, there is no way to stop the fall. What was supposed to be a controlled fall is suddenly out of control. If something as small as a crack can mess someone up, imagine what you could do if you work at it.

Offensive footwork can range anywhere from simply stepping on his foot as you attack to complicated twisting around until you look like a Hindu statue. What they all have in common is that they attack his lower legs and/or his balance—most often both.

In general, I always advise you to go out and play with the concepts you've learned and then reread whatever of my books you got the idea from. See if what I talked about way-back-when has taken on a different perspective. I really advise it in this case. Much in this chapter harkens back to Chapter

5. That is to say, "the reason this works is because of that." And much of what is in this chapter is fine tuning that will make the concepts from that chapter work better.

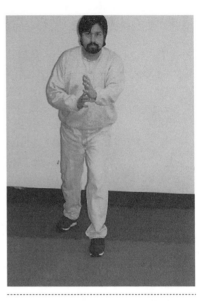
Lead hand and foot change (choo-choo)

I want you to try something. Go stand with your back to a bed and put your feet about a foot out from it. Now step back until your foot runs into the bed. Reset yourself and, *without* moving your feet, shift your body back as if you were stepping backward. The reason for the bed will become immediately obvious. Don't catch yourself, and pay very close attention to where you lost control over gravity. That place is called the "point of no return" (or PNR for short). That is pretty much as far as you have to push someone while standing on his foot to get him to fall. If you follow his body's circle you're going to push him a whole lot farther than that.

As I have said many times already, your goal isn't to fight the guy, it's to climb over him and escape. The very fact that you're using him as traction is going to cause damage. If he falls down in the process, even better.

Imagine what would happen if you took the stomp kick I mentioned last chapter, raked your shoe down his shin, and stomped on his ankle while shoving him down and back with fists and elbows?

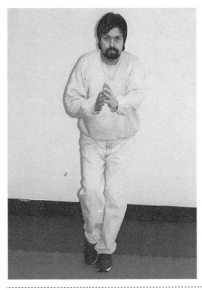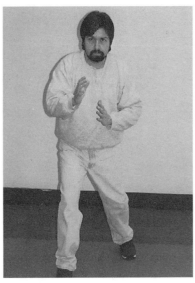

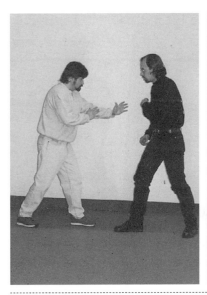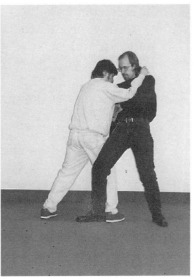

Add to that nailing his foot to the floor so he can't get it out there to save himself. (It's called tripping, and it's a time-honored practice in elementary schools everywhere.)

With a little practice you can easily learn to place your foot where it will act like that crack in the sidewalk, keeping him from re-establishing his balance when you climb over him. Start out with wide inside crescent steps to learn how to come around from his outside, but eventually work your way to just snaking your foot forward and behind his. Now, as much as he wants to back away from you, he can't. This is a form of a throw called a kinjit, and it is a nasty way to fall!

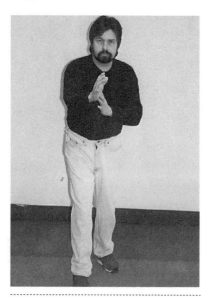

Toe up

Let's look at the unbalanced blitzkrieg wave attack. Like I said, if you block to the outside gate, the attack will be deflected by the wedge. This means he could be like a runaway truck heading past you. Well, you give him a flat and watch the fun. How do you give him a flat? Just stick your foot out as he rushes by you. All of a sudden that foot he so desperately needs to keep from falling is tied up back at the border checkpoint. Oops, STBY!

When he goes rushing by you can whip around with your hands and grab the back of his head, then keep spinning the same direction he's going. Your pull/push will add energy to his headlong flight.

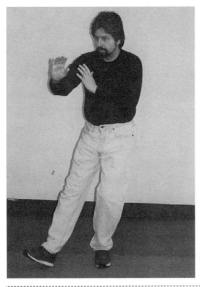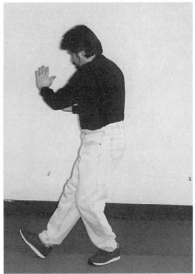

Sound difficult to do? It's just draw the bow and spin the wheel. And remember, sticking your foot out can have major added effect.

You can get a similar effect by grabbing and jerking the guy's arm in the same direction (which is easier to do if you remember to block with an open hand). I'll go into jerks in a bit, but the combination of his forward motion, a jerk, and an inconveniently placed foot can really mess up a guy's day.

With a well-placed foot all sorts of moves can become nearly inescapable. Without that foot many a good takedown will fail. The guy will be able to outrun (or actually out-stumble) the takedown. In doing this, he stays up and remains capable of hurting you. The sooner he hits the ground, the sooner you will be safe.

Anywhere you put your foot next to his can be a stopper. The trick is to always make sure that you're pushing/pulling him against it. In other words, make sure the force you apply makes him step into your foot. That messes up his attempts to keep his balance.

It doesn't matter if you push or pull the guy over your foot; what matters is that you get him moving that way. This is, in effect, a "shearing" action. It's like catching him in a giant pair of scissors. While that may sound complicated, all you are doing is moving him around his circle.

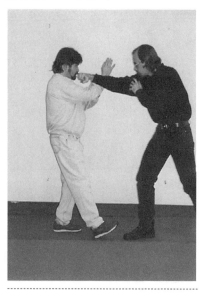

Toe up in action

THE CRANE STRIKE

While I tend to prefer the wing chun jerk (my roots are showing), a bastardized crane strike is an easy beginner's move. The real strike is usually delivered like a shin kick with the wrist. The idea is to clobber someone, but it can be used to move someone as well. This can be done anywhere along your arm, but around the elbow joint seems to have the best effect.

On the opposite side of the direction you want him to go, shoot your arm up and past your opponent like a snake striking (fast and loose), then lock it down as if it's a branch off a tree. Using your body's vertical axis as a pivot, spin the direction you want him to go. I tend to aim for his back, upper chest, or the crook of his neck and shoulders when I do this move.

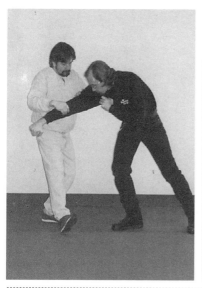
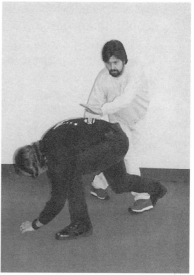

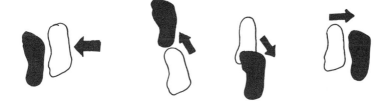

Offensive foot positioning and applied forces (your foot in black)

You can either take him over backward in a clothesline action or shoot him forward. Generally, you will find that doing the forward throw is easier because the footwork is much simpler. All you do is pivot with the toe up. The problem is if you don't get your foot out there (or if there isn't a convenient wall in front of him), he can recover. Don't try to take someone over backward until you've practiced enough to get that foot out there to take him over.

I showed you that move with a straight-in step,

but if you slip to the 45, it lessens your chances of getting hit. Also, the move the guy uses trying to reorient can be used to throw him. He's giving you his body's motion. Factor this movement in, because it will happen.

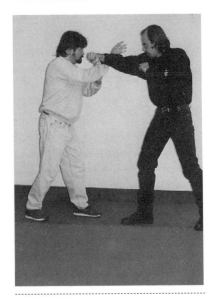

Generally, you want to step to the guy's outside gate even if you have to knock him to the side—which really isn't that hard to do. Snake your hands around his arm as he strikes and move him where you want him. Like I said, just because you leave the centerline for a second doesn't mean you aren't coming back. That A-frame braced wedge block says "MINE!" You get hit less on the outside gate than you do on the inside. It's also much more disorienting for someone when you've moved him like this.

Notice with both this backward takedown and the one before that you are pulling him over your leg from his outside gate. Also notice how the thrower is standing, pulling the guy into his braced stance. This is important to keep from going down with someone you're going to throw.

GOING TO EXTREMES

I'm going to advocate two totally opposite stances with this footwork. Unlike politics, either extreme

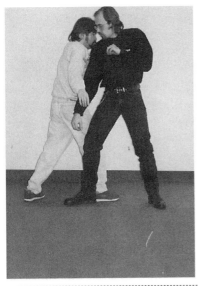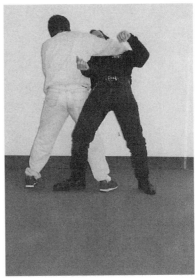

Kinjit (note foot position and opposing force)

works well but the middle of the road will get you squished like a grape. Either put all your weight forward above the leg you are dragging him over (keeping your back leg out there as a brace) or put your weight over the back leg and stick your other, muscle-stiffened leg out there for him to trip over.

This is one of the key elements of offensive footwork. You don't want to distribute your weight evenly over both feet because a balanced stance doesn't handle the person's mass as well as an extreme stance. That's because with a balanced stance you're facing his entire weight with only half of yours. If you try to drag someone over your leg without either putting your weight entirely on it or taking weight off it, odds are you're going to go down with the dude. You might get away with it but it's way more likely you'll end up wrestling.

Let's also talk about stance integrity as another way to keep from going down.[2] You can pull someone into and over your braced stance. The tricky part is not pulling him into you so he can grab you. This is done by moving around your vertical axis, but it helps if you've managed to block and tie up his hands. Otherwise, he can grab onto you as he flies by.

The reason the guy goes over is that his unstable base is pulled over a stable base. See how the force of the guy's body slams into the thrower's braced stance? This kind of move is really good for tight situations where you don't have much room to move. What? You weren't expecting to have to fight between two cars in a parking lot? In a cramped hallway? In a doorway? Kiddies, this is real life, remember?

You'll also notice in all the different ways of doing this that the feet move

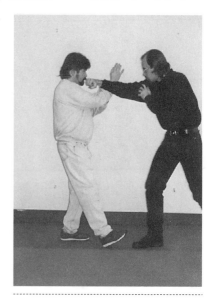

Block

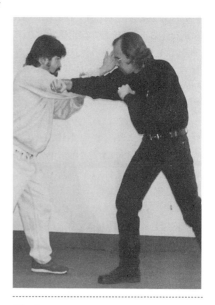

Block

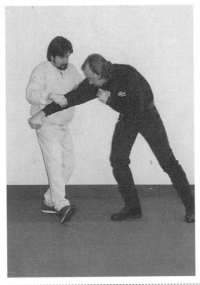

Forward-pull takedown

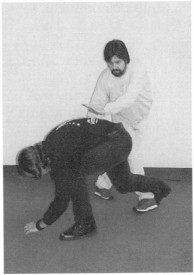

Trip/throw

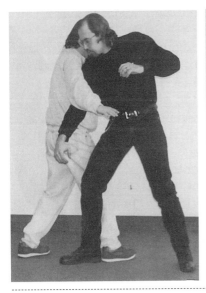

Backward takedown

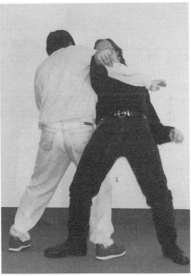

Sweep

Footwork

into position with a step. Face it, you're going to be moving your feet anyway; you might as well be offensive with them.

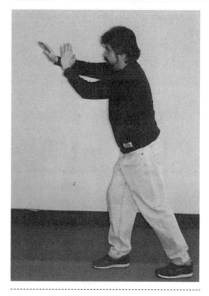

Forward (yes)

Coordinating your feet and hands to move at one time is an incredibly useful skill to learn. I've seen many otherwise effective moves fail when the guy got his hands, but not his feet there. Once again, I recommend going out and getting Stevan Plinck's tape, *Pukalan Pentjak Silat*. It has some incredibly easy ways to learn offensive footwork concepts.

Here is a major point about these kinds of moves that causes people all sorts of trouble (aside from not getting their foot there in time). When you're flapping your arm around to get it into place, most of the motion comes from your arm muscles. But it's better if you relax your arm as you're getting it into place. That gives you speed. Relaxed muscles are fast muscles. Gawd, I'm getting sick of harping on this, but it is so counterintuitive to hard-style martial artist's training that it drives them up the wall. But it is what will make this move either a piece of cake or an unmitigated disaster. Keep your arms relaxed while going out there, then tighten down. The power doesn't come from muscle power; it's coming from your hips and your body's spin.

Now what does this have to do with offensive

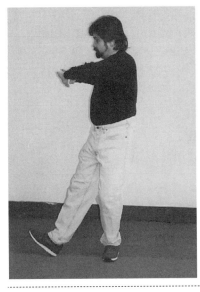 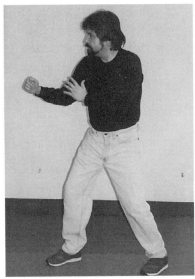

Back (yes)   Evenly divided (no)

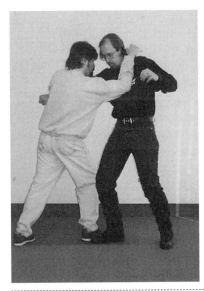 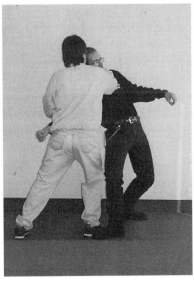

Kinjit into forward stance

footwork? Hold out the shield and walk forward! Better yet, drop step forward. You use your shield arm to act as a conduit of your body's momentum. The fact that you happen to be stepping forward also means you have an opportunity to put your foot in a really annoying place.

THROWS

You may have noticed that the crane strike looks almost like the judo throw. The only difference is that judo and yudo practitioners tend to use their thighs, placed behind their opponent's, to achieve the same effect. Not to belabor the obvious, but it works both ways. The hip-to-hip, knee-to-knee version of this throw is for close-up, while the foot-to-foot crane strike is for a little further back. The principle, however, remains the same.

The advantage in the up-close judo version is that you use your hip to blow his center of balance by dropping below his hips and slamming into him, then whipping him around. This tends to make it a more reliable throw. Even if you use the wrong muscle tension, your body mass can compensate.

The disadvantage is if your opponent catches on that he's falling, he's likely to grab onto the nearest thing to him—better known as you! And he's close enough to get a good hold on you. That means you both go tumbling down. I've seen that happen a lot!

The distance throw tends to prevent mutual takedowns. He's far enough out that he doesn't have anything to grab onto. Even if he tries for your arms, he often can't get a good grip. The disadvantage is that if you don't do it fast enough or get your foot out there, the guy can wiggle out of it by simply jumping back when he realizes something is going wrong. That means you're back where you started, both on your feet and neither having the advantage. This is another reason putting that foot out is so important. It has this nasty habit of preventing him from escaping.

The good news is if he keeps on charging in toward you, he puts himself into the judo throw. Something you should know: If you don't have your muscle tension right (i.e., you're using your hips and body weight instead of upper body strength), both of these moves will turn into a wrestling match. You might have the muscle to get away with it; then again, you might not. Using your body's mass to move him is more reliable than using muscle.

Once you get the hang of the basic move, remember the footwork. Stick a foot out there in the most obnoxious manner possible. I won't go into besets and sapaus, which are a little more complicated, except to say that putting a little extra energy into your tripping foot can give you spectacular results. If you want to see the advanced moves, go get Stevan Plinck's tape. I'm not going to reinvent the wheel.

Here's something that might interest you. With

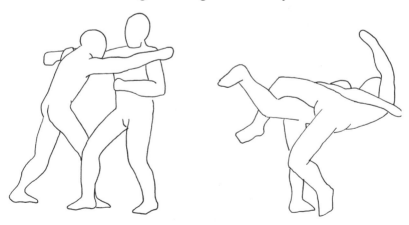

Distance and close

most people power comes from their back foot and back hand. The hand or foot farthest from you will be delivering the major power blows. That's the limb you have to watch for the most damage potential, because the blow coming from there is going to hurt you. Like I said, this is with *most* people. The good news is such moves tend to be slow.

Most people don't know how to throw powerful punches or kicks from their lead leg or hand. Most kicks or punches from the front are just going to be annoyance blows. They'll be fast, but they will do very little damage. EXCEPT, they freak you out! I'm talking Set Ups here. They snake in and slap you; you get nervous about it and go chasing them, thereby leaving yourself open for real hits. Not a good situation.

STANCES

What really confuses me is that most people's fighting stances encourage these kinds of annoyance kicks! Why do you want to do something that not only leaves you open to getting kicked but will stress you out? By stressing out you start making mistakes so a powerful kick can connect. That ain't how we like to do it where I'm from.

Tell me if the next photo looks familiar.

In sports fighting, that is an excellent pose. You can get that front foot off fast for a point. If the guy charges you, all you have to do is rock back and kick. It's a great way to stand if you're looking to rack up points because it opens up all sorts of targets on your opponent.

I'd like to mention, however, that all sorts of things are illegal and off limits in a tournament, even in the most hardcore full-contact pseudo-rumbles. Not so in a real fight. That sports stance presents all sorts of problems in a real fight. The first and foremost is that it is designed to stop the accidental shot to the family jewels. While such moves are off limits in tourneys, accidents do happen. But, of course, there is the cup to protect your social life.

This stance is not real useful against a dedicated attack to the nuggets. That's one place where he doesn't have to hit you hard to make your eyes bug out. Power isn't necessary, but speed is. Stop and think, which kicking foot is closest to the roots of your fantasies? Let me spell it out for you: *the fastest one*!!! You're wide open against an upward roundhouse kick, especially if the guy gets some extra inches by using the ball of his foot.

Are we going "yikes!" yet? Hang on, there's more. The more you stand to the side, the easier it is to break your knee with a side-thrust kick. You may be able to roll away from it in time, but there is a problem: You now have a guy who wants to hurt you standing on your calf, and you're on your knees and facing the other way. A pretty picture this is not. I've achieved the same result many a time by just picking up my foot and doing the stomp kick I told you about to buckle a guy's knee.[3]

Another issue I have with side stances is that they pretty much limit you to moving fast in only one of two ways—forward or backward. You can retreat, but the fastest way to do it is by staying on your opponent's line of orientation. As you now know this means he's got no reason to stop attacking. This stance doesn't let you get offline real fast. It can be done, but not fast and not real gracefully.

But the main problem I have with this stance is that while it is great for kicking, it's seriously weak for the hands. By turning your body sideways, your hands do not go into battle together. One's out flapping in the wind while the other is hanging back doing nothing. It may be hanging back as a second line of defense, but it won't do you any good if it doesn't get out there in time. Moreover, if the front hand gets knocked aside by a blitzkrieg attack, your back-up hand is going to be just as alone facing something that already proved itself strong enough to blast through one hand.

Face it, a weak second line of defense against a charging bull is just as useless as a weak first line. Neither one is going to stop him. The idea is to get your defenses as strong as possible and get them out where they will do you some good in your quest not to get your teeth knocked in.

Understand that I come from forward-facing styles. We cover our cajones by keeping centerline or twisting our hips or getting our blocks down in time. By standing in a forward position we keep both hands out in front at the same time, prevent sweeps, and keep from getting our knees smashed to boot. Slipping off at an angle is easier from this position as well. Oh yeah, we can backpedal faster if something goes wrong, too. Finally, we can twist in either direction to handle whatever is occurring. This is kind of like the stepping forward thing; it begins to make a lot of sense when you know the reasoning behind it.

Most importantly, though, the absolute worst-case scenario when we slip off line is that we end up fighting from a side stance. With a twist of the hips, we're back up front. A front-fighting stance's worst-case scenario is another style's starting point! I've listed the worst-case scenarios from a side-stance position.

I don't expect you to abandon your style's fighting stance for something totally different from what you've trained in. What I would recommend, however, are some modifications. The first thing is that you take care of those pesky front leg kicks. In doing so, you'll protect your social life and really annoy people at tournaments.

Mirror, mirror

Ever look in a mirror and see how things are reversed but not reversed? That's to say the letters in a word will each be reversed, but the entire word is not. This is called mirroring, and it is different than reversal. The standard fighting stance is an out and out reversal (that's what you see in the photo below). Both people put forth their right or both put forth their left. While they increase their chances of scoring with their fast foot, they offer the other guy the same advantage. They are standing with the holes and weaknesses of their stances open to each other. Where I'm from, we call this bad. I want to hit him, not be hit by him.

What I'm going to recommend is that you mirror. That is to say, you reflect back to him with a different side. He sticks out his left side; you stick out your right side. He switches; you switch.

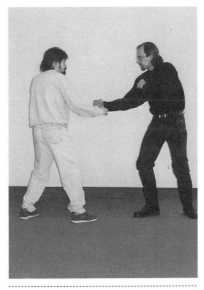

Opposite fighting stance

You can be so annoying with this that it's unbelievable. It will drive kickers absolutely nuts. The reason is that most rely on those fast front-leg kicks for points. By mirroring, you close the door to most of those moves. All of a sudden, unless he can twist himself like a pretzel, that fast leg is facing a blank wall.

Unless he shifts his stance to get opposite to you (in which case you mirror him again), he's going to have to kick with his back leg to get you in the front. That takes longer. Watch for the weight shift onto the front leg, then step forward when he kicks! When he comes around with that kick, you're mirroring him again and you're inside his kick. If he

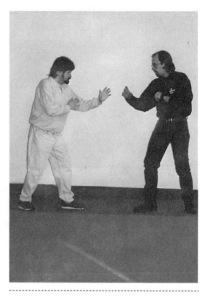

Mirroring

spins around, you're not only on his outside gate, but inside his kick. If he's smart, he'll give up the idea of kicking and back up. If not, well you got a point (or something nastier).

It takes a little practice to get to the point where you automatically mirror the guy's lead back to him, but the rewards are well worth it.

SHIELDS UP

Notice something very minor, but very important. in the photos on page 240 The right hand is forward when the right foot is forward. The left hand is forward when the left foot is forward. This is important for a very simple reason: By presenting a solid side like this, you create a shield. That means anything that is thrown from that side is more than likely to bounce off that shield. It does-

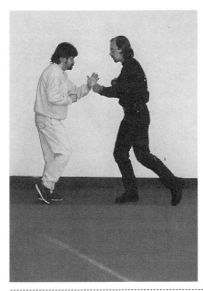
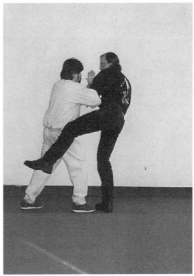

n't matter if it comes in high or low; the shield is out there.

From this position, you have all sorts of options for blocks. The leg-lift block from a previous chapter is a good example. Lift your knee to your elbow and you've created the same block Muay Thai fighters use.

This is such a big shield that it would make a Roman legionnaire gulp in disbelief. Now, squat down and duck your head! You've created a shell and covered all the tourney point areas. Want to swap sides? Step forward or back and stick the same side hand out. Now the other side is shielded.

I want to show you a potential problem here. What happens if you have your left hand and right foot forward?

What you have just done is opened potential holes in your upper right and lower left quadrants. A blow could get through. Now to show what a Machiavellian S.O.B. I am, I'll tell you that this is

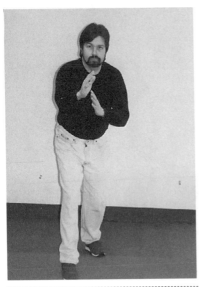 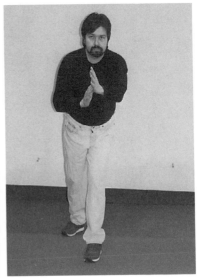

Right/right   Left/left

either a potential problem or a wonderful trap. It's a great way to sucker someone into attacking exactly where you want him to attack. "Yo, step inta mah crib," said the spider to the fly.

LET'S DO LUNGE

One more thing I'd like to address: do you step or lunge to move in any direction? The answer is, it depends. Learn both. They both have offensive and defensive applications.

A quick rundown is that a lunge keeps whatever foot is forward, forward. A step changes leads. That should help you differentiate between the two. Although, just to muddy up the water, the drop step can be done as either a lunge or a step.

I learned the lunge when I was studying fencing.[4] The secret to a lunge is that you basically jump into a fall. You coil your rear leg or you stand

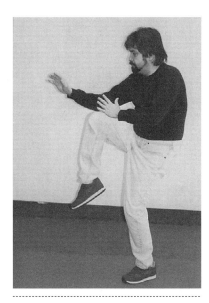

Muay Thai block/shield

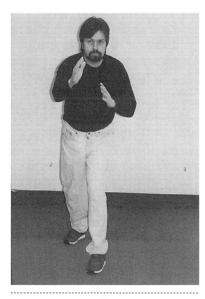

Don't do this unless it's a trap

with it coiled. You lift your lead foot and as you begin to fall, you spring off that coiled leg. As your body drops, you catch yourself with your front foot.

What I'm showing on the next page is a fencing lunge. It is far too extreme to be of any real use in a fight, but by practicing it you can more easily understand how it can work in less pronounced versions.

Unlike in an actual fencing lunge, you will not leave your rear foot dangling out there. Once you've shoved off, drag it back underneath you as a brace, coiled to spring again.

By dropping your body weight in this manner you, in effect, do a drop step. Your entire body mass starts moving courtesy of gravity and is then sped up by your muscles. Go out and

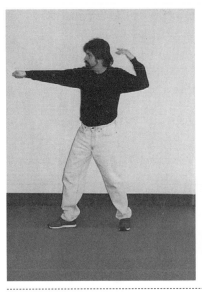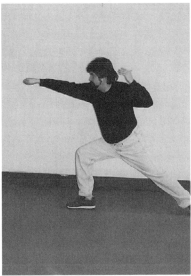

Fencing lunge

practice this move until you can do it in its
extremes, then begin to work on it in smaller and
smaller versions. Try to get it down to where you
can do it within a foot.

The next thing is to practice lunging in different
directions. Do everything from "straight ahead" all
the way around to "straight back." Cover all 360
degrees. The trick to making all of this easier (and
faster) is that you actually direct the way you're
going by moving your hips. Lift a leg, shift your center of balance in that direction, then push off with
your other leg.

A lunge allows you to cover a lot of area in very
little time. But it can also allow you to plow into
someone with your shield. Brace up your wedge and
lunge into him on either side of his centerline and
you'll send him spinning—especially if he's in the
middle of a blitzkrieg attack.

At the very least, you're going to send him spin-

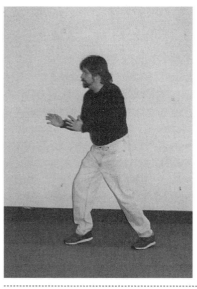
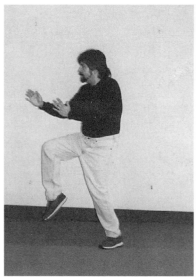

Fighting lunge

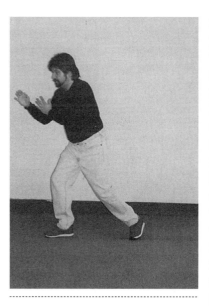

ning. If you decide to place your foot somewhere special (we covered that already, remember?), odds are he's going to fall down. Remember, after you've slammed into him with your body weight, you speed him along his way by pointing to where you want him to fall using your arm muscles. Isn't it neat the way it all ties back together?

A step changes

your lead. One use for this is when the guy realizes that he can't come in on you with a fast annoyance blow (because you're mirroring him) and he tries to throw a slower, more powerful kick from his back leg. Well, guess what? As he comes in, you step forward and change leads. You mirror! So what if he's throwing a blow? You're putting your shield out there to block it. Add to that you're

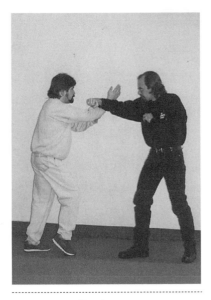

Lunge in application

moving off the range of his blow and running into him at the same time!

From this new position you're able to do all sorts of things from hits to throws to body checks to elbows in really tender spots. The only limit is your imagination. If you keep firmly in mind that your main goal is to get out of there, then the "best" move will automatically present itself.

By the way, to learn to shift leads with your hands, pretend you're an old steam locomotive. Actually, you're more like a kid playing choo-choo. Lead hand drops, rear hand comes over. Former lead hand retracts to rear centerline position. Mix it with a step, and you can go "chugga-chugga-chugga-chug" all over the dojo. I'll warn you in advance, you'll get some seriously weird looks if you do the whistle sound, too.

In case you hadn't noticed, the stance that I've

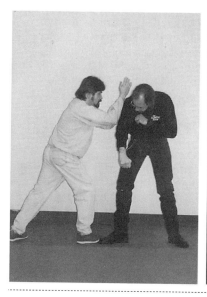 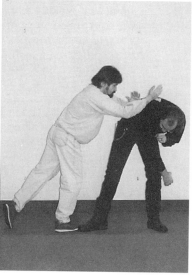

been showing you here has one really important advantage. It's an instinctive stance for when someone takes an unexpected swing at you. Think about it: What do you do when suddenly attacked? Step back and put your hands up, right? Well, this just refines it. Instead of getting your hands up just any old which way, you bring them up on centerline while stepping back. This creates the block, as well. Unlike most martial arts, you're not stepping back into a stance. Your block is your stance and your stance is your block. They happen at the same time.

Pretty slick, huh?

Wait until you get to the point where you automatically step forward into this stance. That's when the fun really starts!

---

[1]   As a point of instruction, many women do not consciously recognize that a blow to a man's chest is nowhere near as

painful as it would be to a woman. Guys have nothing to squish, yet many women aim blows there. These blows would, to another woman, be extremely painful, but they have no effect on a man. If you are teaching self-defense, making women aware of this physiological difference is important.

[2] Stance integrity is the imaginary line between your feet. We have a stable base along this line and can resist pressure from either side. However, any force that hits us perpendicular to this line has a tendency to knock us on our butts. If you watch two guys who have clinched, you will see that they usually go down when one or the other manages to push/pull in a perpendicular manner.

[3] You will find that styles that allow legs as targets tend to take a more forward stance, for a variety of good reasons. Take a lesson from the folks who get attacked this way.

[4] I studied saber. What can I say, I like chopping my enemies into little pieces. Fencing is also great for annoying kendoists. But if you really want to put their panties in a wad, come at them with broadsword and shield. That pretty much torques everyone's wa. Everyone touts Oriental swordplay, but Westerners were no slouches at the old choppity-chop themselves. It's just that honkies discovered more effective ways to kill each other.

More Low-Down, Dirty Tricks

*The purpose of a warship is to bring the
maximum amount of aggravation possible
to the enemy . . .*

—Dick Nelson

In case you haven't noticed, my intent with this
book has been to keep you from getting your face
pushed inside-out.

Most books on making martial arts street effective go on and on about how to tear your attackers'
faces off. They tend to ignore small little details,
such as you're probably right in the middle of an
ambush when the subject comes up.

As a streetfighter, I know something that most
martial artists don't: I can get my ass kicked if I
don't pay attention to what my opponent is doing.
That's why I wanted to cover keeping you safe,
first. It's now time to make sure that your opponent
ends up feeling like he crawled through a barbed-
wire fence to fight a bobcat in a briar patch. At last,
we turn our attention to ripping off his face.

When I was a kid, people used to say to me,

"You fight like a girl." I was a firm believer in scratching, biting, pulling hair, and pinching. When I grew up and perfected my craft, my opponents realized that it wasn't a girly-girl way of fighting. Much to their horror they realized I fought like my namesake: an animal. I clawed, I bit, I gouged, I headbutted, I choked, I swatted, I crushed, I tore. There was nothing so low-down and vicious that I didn't do it. In other words, I did everything I could in order to be the last man standing.

Guess what? This mano-a-mano, stand-there-toe-to-toe-and-punch-each-other stuff is probably the stupidest way there is to fight. Granted, it looks good on TV. But real life is not about how it looks; it's about staying out of the hospital. Your purpose is to damage him and, in doing so, keep him from doing it to you first. That not only means doing unto him before he can do unto you, but using every rotten, low-down, sneaky trick and advantage to guarantee you'll win. Because that's exactly what he is going to do to you. If he didn't have something nasty up his sleeve that he thought would guarantee him victory, he wouldn't be there in the first place! So if you want to live long enough to lie to your grandkids, let's take that manly-man, mano-a-mano, fair-play, toe-to-toe slug-out concept and chuck it out the window.

We generally decry people who cheat at cards. Such a person is taking unfair advantage of those who abide by the rules. Only one person cheating (or maybe two working together) can really take unfair advantage of innocents. Of course, if everyone at the poker table is cheating, you got yourself one hell of an interesting game. (Just how many aces is a deck of cards supposed to have again?) It's no longer poker, it is a balls-to-the-wall free-for-all that only looks like poker. Now all of a sudden we are back to skill being the determining factor. It becomes a matter of who's the better cheater.

And that is exactly what a streetfight is. It's a contest to determine who's the dirtier fighter. The guy you're up against came to the table thinking that he was the only one who could cheat. He's got the deck stacked against you. Odds are, he's bringing a few extra buddies, a couple of dirty tricks, or maybe even a weapon to ensure he wins. But how was he to know that you're just as willing and able to break the rules as he is?

Let me give you the biggest bucket of ice water there is to toss on would-be troublemakers. As long as you are both playing inside the rules, fine and dandy, but when he steps out, you step out too. Stepping outside the rules is not the sole domain of anyone. I used to love to listen to criminals whine and complain that the police had set them up. They honestly thought breaking the rules was their special right. Sorry sucker, that ain't the way it works. By stepping outside the rules you run the risk that you might have company out there. And all them nice cushy rules to keep people from getting hurt no longer apply to either party. By the way, you might want to keep this in mind before you decide to get froggy about the rules, too.

The biggest deterrent is when the guy looks at you and realizes you will move outside the rules just as fast as he will. All of a sudden, the advantages he gains by taking it there dry up faster than a politician's promise. It all comes back to win, lose, or draw, he'll be hurting. With this in mind, let's look at how to make him say "Oww!"

A major misconception is that the best way to inflict damage on someone is through impact. It only takes one viewing of the Rodney King tape to see that you can seriously whomp on someone and it won't stop him. Say whatever else you like about it, but impact techniques didn't stop him. If four big cops with tonfas can't stop one pissed-off drunk, what makes you think hitting one with your fist is going to do all that much?

Let's take a long and hard look at impact-style training. Whether you agree with it or not, I highly recommend you sit down and think about what I am about to say. I want to reiterate: The guy you are sparring with is not an enemy. You're not going full force and hitting him with everything you have.[1] There is always that tendency to pull punches and then think, "Well, if I'd hit him with everything I had it would have stopped him."

Unless you've actually had to hit someone to stop him, how do you know what would or wouldn't stop a person? You don't.

How hard you have to hit someone to stop them depends entirely on how much he is willing to suffer to get you. The more he's willing, the harder you have to hit. I've gone up against some tough hombres in my life, and I can tell you that size is seldom the determining factor. I've had little guys take blows that dropped gorillas twice their size, and I've had big guys just look at me after I gave them my best shot. I will tell you that some of the hardest, most brutal fights I have ever been in have been against guys my own size or smaller (granted there ain't that many smaller, but they do exist). Let me tell you that size is irrelevant when the guy is committed to taking your head off.

The other determining factor of how much pain and damage you have to inflict is the threat level. Someone who brings a weapon or buddies with him has just bumped his status up to "high threat level." His ability to do greater damage and do it faster makes it so. That is someone I am going to hit with everything I have to stop him before he can do damage to me. You don't have time to waste hoping that a minor strike will convince him to back off. Such a blow will only convince him to shoot or will convince his buddies to attack en masse. By choosing to cheat in this manner, laughing boy has ensured the kid gloves are off.

In the dojang (and even the ring), there is an aversion to doing things that would cripple your opponent. The guy is not your enemy and you're not trying to disable him.[2] Therefore you don't tend to normally think of smashing knees, gouging out eyes, or crushing throats as regular moves. Don't think this doesn't affect what you expect when you go into a fight.

Want to know just a few things you might have to do out there? Or worse yet, face having done to you? In my time, I've picked up and dribbled a guy on a pool table before he could knife me, crawled all over guys to get out the door before their buddies got me, slammed a trash can over a gang member's head, busted pool cues across people's faces, smashed a beer mug into a guy's face and threw him into his buddies, head butted, busted knees, gouged out eyes, and ripped ears—I even stabbed a guy before he could shoot me. These are the realities of what it takes to survive a streetfight. If the guy I was up against didn't bring the commitment to endure these things in order to get me, he lost.

Most people only bring with them the commitment to hurt you. They don't want to get hurt themselves, but they are more than willing to hurt you, sometimes even kill you. I once read, "A bully doesn't want to fight you, he wants to beat you up and be done with it." That's pretty true from all that I have seen. If the guy thinks he can get away with hurting you with little to no damage to himself, he will get froggy.

More Low-Down, Dirty Tricks

What I'm trying to say here is that most people who pick fights don't have the dedication to keep on coming at you if they are getting hurt. They don't want to play anymore. They tend to pick up their marbles and go home. I say this after having gone head to head with some of the baddest of the bad—gang members, psychos, trained killers, and all sorts of other charming individuals.

Most of these yahoos think they're going to cause you all sorts of damage and just walk off. This is especially true of career criminals or gang members. They are punks. They don't expect to get back what they are willing to give.[3] Of all the people you're likely to end up in conflict with, these clowns most closely resemble the bully statement. They usually bring along weapons and numbers and have no hesitation about using them to hurt you without getting hurt themselves.

This is why, in any criminal confrontation, the goal GET OUT OF THERE stands above all else. If you think you're going to stand around and fight them off, that delusion is going to last until one of them successfully deploys a weapon. Then you're either dead or in the hospital. *Do not try to stand around and spar!* The longer you stay there, the better his chances of successfully using his weapon.

Another barrel of laughs is the clown who thinks he's invincible, so he goes out and looks for fights. Any reason will do to start one. This is the guy who jumps in your face for just breathing. Going back to that fight in the movie *Dazed and Confused*, that tough guy is a good example. He jumps in the other kid's face for a passing comment.

This moron thinks he can soak up a few hits as he charges in on you. And in light of the way most people throw ineffective punches, he's right. What makes him a pain in the butt is that this delusion of

Taking It to the Street

invincibility makes him super aggressive. Add to that he has the experience of doing this kind of stuff and getting away with it.

I will tell you right now these guys will freak out your little monkey brain because they get up on you for no reason. There you are minding your own business one second, and BAM! next second this snarling, drooling attitude is up in your face. That's where most people go, "Huh?" and freak out. They are not used to unexpectedly dealing with this intense aggression. Before they can figure out what to do other than say, "homina, homina, homina," the jerk is all over them.[4]

The other thing you're going to run into is someone whose emotional state has overwhelmed his rational mind. Whether from alcohol, drugs, or just extreme circumstances, the person's emotions are running the boat. It's what Goleman calls an "emotional hijacking." Such people are so blinded by what is going on inside their own heads that they are neither rational nor aware of reality. The bad news is that when they move, they move with the same suicidal commitment as a gangbanger.[5]

The thing with any of these scenarios is that their main idea is to hurt you while avoiding getting hurt themselves. The door swings both ways—they can get hurt too. Once they start hurting, most get all flustered and hairless. It's no longer any fun. It's no longer the easy way to win. This is especially true if they start getting hurt in unexpected ways.

It's a rare individual who will knowingly sacrifice himself to get to you. I will, however, tell you that the guy you have to worry the most about is the dude who knows that you'll get a serious piece out of him and yet is dedicated enough to still keep coming in to take you out. That is and always has been the difference between a punk and a pro. A pro, knowing the price, will have made a conscious decision to still come on. A punk will get hairless when things don't go the way he planned and he starts getting hurt. I'll go into the realities of this kind of person more in the next chapter, but let me tell you right now that they do exist, and in large numbers.

The good news is that seldom do these types actively go out looking for trouble. Or if they do, they are only in certain areas that the wise steer clear of. The bad news is that if you bring it to them . . . well, they are the bad news.

The reason I took this weird side trip has to do with what I call the "judo-syndrome." Mind you, I am an advocate of judo. On several occasions, however, I have seen a moron attack and be thrown by a judoka. THE IDIOT THEN GETS UP AND ATTACKS AGAIN! The reason is simple—numb nuts thinks he slipped! He gets up madder than a wet hen because now, on top of everything else, he's lost face. He doesn't realize that the guy he's facing is a trained fighter, who *chose* not to hurt him! Nope, until something breaks through that thick skull, he's going to keep on coming. What will break through is pain and disorientation.

I'll let you in on a major fighting secret. There are different types of pain, and a person who is expecting one type will most often be unnerved by another type. While there are people who can "take" certain types of pain and keep on coming, there are very few people who are true "horses" (someone who can endure incredible pain of almost any type).

A good example of this is the reaction some people have to pepper spray. There are people who can withstand it. You'll spray them and they will keep on coming. This is one of the boogeyman stories that folks selling self-defense classes tell. "Eeek! Freak! The spray you were expecting to protect you doesn't work!" Better go out and take this guy's class.[6]

OK, so let me get this straight—since the guy is expecting the pain of the pepper spray, he can brace himself against it and keep on going. And that proves what? That someone who is expecting a certain type of pain can keep on coming through it, or that, as the self-defense teacher claims, pepper sprays are useless? I dunno, Einstein. I think it's time for some scientific peer review here.

What if I kick him in the nuts first and THEN spray him? Would he still be able to take it and keep on coming? Or would the different types of pain not allow him to function? Would an unexpected type of pain distract him from his braced "I'm ready for this kind of pain" mind-set and, in doing so, make the first type of pain effective again? (Oddly enough, none of these spray-proof studs have ever offered to prove me wrong on this one. Hmmm, I wonder why?) I know humans can resist one force at a time, but I also know that two at once, and from unexpected directions, tend to mess them up. Betcha that works here, too.

Figure the guy coming at you is expecting a certain type of pain. Odds are he's banking on you to throw a few ineffective punches before he overwhelms you and starts waltzing on your face. Guess what? You're going to give him all sorts of new definitions of pain. And in ways that will make him wish he had died as a child.

Realize that many of the moves you'll learn in this book have something in common with t'ai chi. T'ai chi is, in my opinion, martial arts with the horns and claws taken off. While most of what I've shown you has been from the defensive aspect, it doesn't take a whole lot to put the sharp edges

back on and get something really effective and brutally offensive.

Something as minor as how you position your
arm when you step forward can spell the difference
between a snowplow-like pushing force and a gor-
ing bull. An open hand can arrive like a snake slid-
ing gently over a surface or a wet towel plopping
down or a grizzly bear paw that crushes, rends, and
claws that same surface. How well you know all the
different levels determines how well you can cheat.
It can get real nasty, real quick, and in all sorts of
different ways.

What we're going to address is how to make
attacking you real painful. It's no longer just a matter
of keeping the guy from hitting you, it's making sure
he is so busy hurting that he doesn't get up and
come after you. There is no judo syndrome; he's
going to know the reason he is hurting is no accident.

Repeating myself again, the human body is like a
suit of armour. It's got its hard spots and its chinks.
Without these chinks, we wouldn't be able to move.
Learn these areas and practice accuracy. One well-
placed blow can do the work of 10 poorly placed
strikes of the same strength. You will only have time
for about three—make them do the work of 30.

Put chunks of tape on your heavy bag and AIM!
Never throw a blow without a 1-inch spot as your
target. When you throw a kick or a punch in the air,
aim for an imaginary target. If you don't have a bag,
put spots on the walls and practice poking at them
with your fingertips to improve your accuracy.

Being able to hit the chinks earns bonus points.
Being struck here hurts more, and it affects his structure and ability to move. The guy summed it up perfectly in the movie *Roadhouse*: "No matter how big
the guy is, if you take his knee out, he goes down."
That's true. That's just one example of a major chink.

But if you don't aim for the fish's eye[7] when you practice, you won't be able to hit a target under stress. What good is knowing that you need to take out his knee if you can't hit it? Much of what I will say from here on depends on your being able to get your hands, knees, or elbows to specific spots. Learning this sort of accuracy is your responsibility, and I know of no other way than practice.

I recommend you get ahold of my book *Fists, Wits, and a Wicked Right* for a rundown on various blows and where to apply them for the most effect. See if you can find a class on pain point compliance technique (PPCT). If nothing else, go find an old Bruce Tegner book, such as *Self-Defense Nerve Centers and Pressure Points for Karate, Jujitsu and Atemi-Waza.* It doesn't matter where you get the information, but getting it is really important.

Incidentally, another training point is to perfect what you know. To this day, I will stand there and practice the same blow, over and over and over again. I will do entire workouts throwing nothing but elbows; another, open-hand strikes; another, knees, etc. Having three moves that you can do accurately, quickly, and powerfully is worth 100 moves that you can only do piss-poorly. Find a move that is repeated again and again in your kata. Then practice it alone and learn how to do it perfectly. Not only does it give that move power and speed, but it makes your katas better.

Now that I've been off into training la-la land, let's get back into kicking some butt. Impacts rely on a forward motion slamming into something. A blow moving down a line (or angle) crashes into a target. This is the basis for most hard styles of martial arts—your blow literally slams into your opponent.

Understand, however, that same motion can be reversed with the same amount of power. When you reverse a move, instead of slamming into your opponent with a push, you jerk him with a pull.

Take a normal hook punch. Instead of just punching and stopping, open your hand and imagine you're grabbing something. With the same force as your punch, jerk back along the same line. If you had his arm, shoulder, or the back of his head, what would that do to him? Either he will just flat-out fall, or he'll chicken-dance to keep from falling. If you grab ahold of something real tender and do this, it hurts like a mother. Even if it doesn't tear off that tender vittle, he's still going to be doing the funky chicken to stay upright. That buys you time, no matter what happens.

Your open hands can be like giant lobster claws. Nothing they glom onto is going to get away. You can either push or pull and he will follow (maybe not willingly), because what you grab will either follow or get torn off. Imagine someone grabbing your nuts and then trying to shot-put them across the room. Now you're getting the idea.

This is not something hard or sport styles do. Their entire focus is on that forward impact. The return motion is not used to further the attack. In doing this, they throw away half of their opportunity to bring grief to their opponents. Your returning action is more than just getting into place where you can attack again. It, too, can be an attack! This constant attack isn't a "high belt" issue; this is something you need to start doing from day one.

If you learn how to do this you will have doubled your attacks. No longer will your backward motion be wasted. Instead of attack, withdraw, attack, withdraw, it becomes attack, attack, attack, attack! What hurts more—Fluffy digging his claws in or tearing them out? Silly question, they both hurt!

The main ingredient of any of these moves is

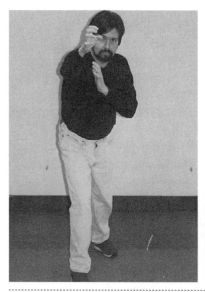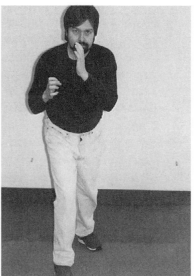

Jerk and rip

hand strength. It's time to start squeezing tennis balls. If you want, you can go out and get any of the many different hand exercisers. But you can play fetch with your dog and give yourself foot massages with tennis balls, which makes them more useful as well as cheaper. If nothing else, go out and grab handfuls of dirt and squeeze. Whatever you choose, crush it, grip it, pinch it, and drive your fingers into it. Learn to clamp down as well as drive your fingers into soft tissue. Become both Larry the Lobster and Fluffy the Cat.

While fingers digging in hurt, it's their coming out that causes the most damage. The easiest way to explain how to do this is that it is literally a punch in reverse. The same motion you do outward to punch, do coming back. Like a punch, the more body weight you put behind it, the better.

As a general point of reference, when you do a jerk to drag someone off balance, you want to pull down toward the ground, pointing to where you want him to fall. When you do a rip, pull back toward yourself and chamber for another attack.

Here's another freebie on how to do arm jerks effectively. Grab his upper arm and pull in the direction it is pointing. Naturally, you're going to add a downward motion to that, but if the guy's arm is pointing out to the side, pull to the side. If it's pointing forward, pull forward. Obviously, when I say pull forward I don't mean pull him into you, but rather pull him to either side of you.

There are all sorts of reasons why this works best (just as there are all sorts of reasons why trying to do it another way will turn it into a hairball). Basically, by just pulling in whatever direction his upper arm is pointing you get an immediate connection to his body weight and balance. If you try to point that upper arm in a different direction first, he'll catch on that you're up to something and have time to resist you. So while technically you can pull it in other directions and grab him by the wrist and pull him down, you'd have to do six other things first. Those are entirely too complicated and are functionally useless in the real thing without 20 years of training. The simple rule of thumb is to follow the upper arm. It's easier and more bulletproof.

Jerks are done with your entire body weight. Whether you grab, lock down, and spin the wheel all the way to the ground, or grab and draw the bow until the very last second, when you crank it into a short, sharp spin the wheel, getting your body weight into it at some time is important.[8]

Rips are what I call "maimers." Since I first mentioned them in *Cheap Shots* back when the earth's crust was still cooling, I've had a lot of people ask me how to do them. Well, you can spend years learning and still not know all the different ways.

However, there is a quick and simple formula. First off, think of muscles as slabs of rock. When you want to pick up a flagstone, how do you do it? You don't grab right in the middle. You find the edge of the slab, wrap your fingers around it and lift.

Same thing with maimers. Find the edge of the muscle, dig your fingers in around and behind it, and pull. Maimers are aimed at the edge of muscles and behind them.

Right now, reach up and grab your chest muscle. Stick your fingers into the middle of your pectoral muscle and try to dig in. Not much happening there is it? Now, put your fingers where your pectoral muscle meets with your chest (under your armpit and slightly to the front). Flex your chest—feel where the muscle connects? Now relax your chest muscle. Dig your fingers into this seam and pinch as if you were about to pick up a rock slab. Now imagine what would happen if you jerked back real hard. Ugly, neh?

If you've ever had a strained tendon or pulled a muscle, you know what you are about to do to the guy with this move. Where ever there is a slab of muscle or a seam between muscles that you can get your hands around, you have a place to do a maimer.

Anywhere there is a bone protuberance that you can hook your fingers behind is also a prime spot—the bottom of the rib cage, the collar bone, the orbital sockets, or the back of the jaw. Anywhere you can dig your fingers behind, hook, and then pull can be used.

In the same vein, anything that is sticking out on the body is a prime target: lips, ears, genitals, all can be grabbed and ripped. The nose can be used, too; however, its prime susceptibility is to upward motions. Open-palm strikes to the snot locker do catch people's attention, believe me. (Don't worry about driving his nose into his brain; that's pretty much a myth.[9]) Following up such a strike by digging your fingers into his eyes will make him reconsider the wisdom of attacking you.

I would now like to address something that people just flat out don't expect. I've said before that every streetfighter worth his salt expects an attempted kick to his nuts. HOWEVER, what men don't expect is a grab to the same place. It's one of those psychological things that people just don't do! I mean, hey, when was the last time a total stranger just walked up and grabbed you by the crotch? Unless you're a male stripper, that just don't happen!

While a rising knee is an immediate danger signal, a downward-shooting hand isn't! For some squirrely reason it doesn't register on the radar. Go out and rent the movie *Sunset* with James Garner, and you'll see how well it works to catch someone's attention. What is most amazing is how freaked out men get when you try to twist off their testicles. I mean even if you miss, they back away real quick saying, "I may want to reconsider messing with this guy!" But then again, you lay a dragon swat onto someone's gonads and he's going to have things on his mind other than thinking you're a pervert.[10]

Moving on any soft flesh that you can dig your fingers into is also a prime target. This includes body fat. With some guys you can't reach their muscles through all the blubber, but you can try to rip their skin off. Dig in and rip. A subtle variation is holding your hand spread out wide when you strike to do this. In doing so, you gather in as much flesh as you can. The rest is your standard rip.

One of my most favorite maimer blows is the dragon. It is a combination of a strike and a maimer, and it has about eight different levels of ugly to it. Many hard stylists are familiar with the strike called the bear swat (or bear paw). Well, the bear is a warm fuzzy version of the dragon. They took the claws off.

First we have your basic bear swat. If the style you study doesn't have a bear swat, find someone whose style does and have him teach you how to do it. If your style does have them, ask your instructor to show you. You may have to listen to a spiel about it being an advanced technique, yada, yada, yada. Great, now will you teach me?

The difference between a bear swat and a dragon is that while both hit with the palm, the bear curls the fingers up—which makes them useless. The dragon, in pulling the fingers back, has five switchblades waiting to pop out after you hit. Your fingertips don't stick out past the flat of your palm. When you hit, the claws extend and dig in (and sometimes grab). Then you rip your way out.

The fat guy variation is that the claws are spread really wide so they can grab and pinch a hunk of flesh. Keeping your fingers together allows you to dig into muscle and bone protuberances more easily, while the wider claw allows for a better grip into soft tissue.

Go out and practice slamming your hands into a heavy bag and digging your fingers in. The action is

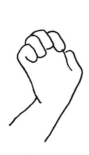   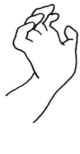   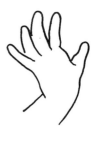

Bear   Dragon   Fat guy

swat, dig in, rip out. As you rip away, your finger-nails should make a scraping sound on the canvas of the bag. If you don't have a heavy bag, try a duffel bag filled with clothes. If all else fails, your bed's mattress will do.[11]

Finally, to remove any doubt about me being a vicious S.O.B., remember that sweeping crane strike thing I showed you in Chapter 10 ("Footwork")? It's real interesting if while your maimer has him doing the funky chicken toward you, that sweep comes out and shears him back the other way. With what you know now, the very thought of this should have you cringing.

Moving on, we get into Br'er Bear fu. While it may sound like I'm down on impact, I'm not. I just believe in making sure that impacts are severe enough to cause major interruption to the guy's sys-tems.[12] When you hit, hit hard and in a vital spot. If your blow doesn't meet that criteria, don't bother throwing it. That kind of blow won't stop your attacker, and there's only limited time before the guy lands on your face. In that limited time, what do you want to throw—three effective blows or three annoyance blows?

Believe it or not, you can hit harder with your palm. Not only does it lessen the chances of your breaking your hand when you hit, but—by removing the wrist as a possible shock absorber—it enables you to hit harder. More force is going into your opponent than is being bled off into space. Don't be fooled by the apparent softness; it's that sumo wrestler thing again.

How do you do this strike most effectively? Look at your watch. Tighten your muscles and spin around your vertical axis. For a straight shot, spin around your vertical axis and pretend your elbow is being thrown off a rolling ball. As you pivot, it shoots out and tightens down just before impact. I told you the stuff you knew already could have horns put on it. Go out and pound on a heavy bag this way for 20 minutes and see how far you can chase the sucker.

There also is an added benefit when you hit like this in the face. With a flip of your wrist, your open hand lands over his eyes. It's really disorienting to have someone's hand land over your face like a face-hugger from the *Alien* movies. That's if you don't just dig your fingers into his eyes.

This brings up a very neat concept and an even neater move. I've heard this move called many things. It is well known in silat and kuntao, but Peyton Quinn gave it its most easily understood name: "The Alien."

Quite literally, you can take the guy down with your fingertips. Of course the fact that your fingertips are being backed up with your entire body weight crawling over him makes it all the more effective. You can twist and turn him in all sorts of neat ways. From this position it's real easy to take him along his circle.

To start with, where his head goes his body will follow. Second, his head and neck are on his vertical axis, and they are the farthest point on his horizontal axis. Third, while his body may be able to resist your force, his neck muscles won't. Finally, there is the natural reaction to pull one's face away from a hand being placed on it. That puts him right where you want him, at the edge of his cone of balance. All of these combine to give you a mini-gyroscope to control the big one.

I'm going to direct you to Bob Orlando's books and videos for fine-tuning this kind of move. From him I learned the best description of how your hand should land on the guy's face—it's like a wet towel.

You plop your hand down like the wet dishrag you used to lob at your sister. Then you just snake your hand around as if you're wiping off a bowling ball; your fingertips and palm start the guy's head around his circle. Once you've wiped, tighten down your muscles and step forward—that puts your body weight onto his head. Now, just point where you want him to go. (Remember, down, not over yonder.)

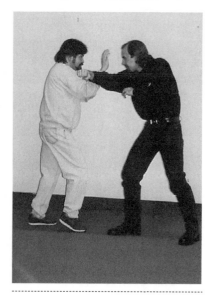

The Alien in action

I have noticed that larger and stronger people have an easier time taking the victim backward over his horizontal axis. Their superior size and strength often compensate for less-than-perfect technique. They just reach out and grab, then shove. (Insert mandatory nagging about relying on muscle.) If, however, you are not a gorilla, you might find that first rolling the person's head to the side works better. You're still going introduce him to terra firma, but that side spin before taking him over the horizontal axis makes the whole thing a little bit easier. Like I said, go out and get Bob Orlando's tapes on this stuff. He gives excellent explanations.

Anyway, back to impacts. Part of the reason I like infighting is because so few people do it well. There are a lot of grapplers out there who, if they get their hands on you, can make your life miserable. In the same vein there are loads of people out

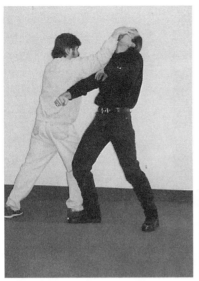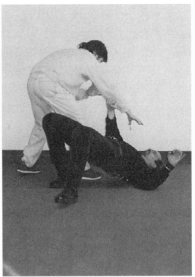

there who will blast you into the next state if you try to hang back. Infighters, however, like up close and personal, but they really aren't interested in hugging anybody like grapplers are. One of the favorite weapons of infighters is the elbow.

There are a couple of ways to throw elbows. While there are better ways, I'll tell you to throw them like you would a uppercut—that is to say, from the hips. Stick your elbows out and twist. Use your vertical axis and hips. Drive into his body with your elbow as if you're trying to plant it into his vertical axis. Wearing a long-sleeved shirt, go after a heavy bag. Shoot elbow strikes into the bag from the side. From the front, put your elbow on the swing again.

Again, aim for the spots of tape, but when you hit them, drive into the bag. You're aiming at its vertical axis—that's where your blow stops. Don't try to push through the bag. Driving through your target is a breaking technique. With such a blow, if the guy is not solidly rooted, all you end up doing is pushing him back. On the other hand, if you aim any blow at his vertical axis, the entire force of the blow goes into his body, whether he is rooted or not. Guess which one hurts more?

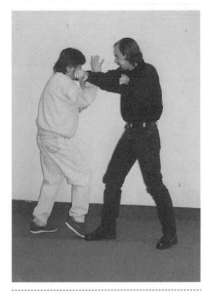

Side-swipe Alien

The reasons I recommend working heavily with elbows are threefold. One, it is incredibly easy to deliver all your body weight into such a blow. Elbow shots can easily be the Nighty Nite Bunny Rabbit strike of a fight—especially if they land in the guy's face as he's rushing past, having just fallen off your wedge. Even if they just hit a slab of muscle/armour, they hurt! Two, elbows are not only hard, but sharp. They focus the force of your blow (and your body weight) into a small, hard, and nasty area. Third, and most important, as you're climbing over the guy, they keep him from getting a good hold on you by pile-driving into his tender spots. Trust me I've taken enough elbows in my life to know that they are way worse than almost any punch and most kicks. They hurt.

I hope by now you're beginning to see why someone who goes into a fight thinking only of punching and kicking is sorely limited. There are literally thousands of other things you can do. Not

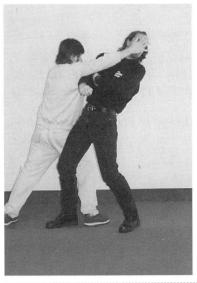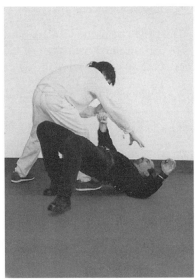

Side-swipe Alien landing.

only do they come in unexpected ways, but they hurt in other unexpected ways, too. Someone who is expecting a punch will jump and yelp when unexpectedly burned by a cigarette.

In a great many ways someone who comes to a situation thinking that his weapon will do all the work for him is in the same boat. His weapon's effectiveness far exceeds that of punches and kicks. Anyone who tries to best him in that manner will lose. But how effective is his weapon going to be when it is brushed aside and he is unexpectedly picked up and slammed headfirst into the sidewalk? Even if that doesn't stop him, by the time he picks himself up and reorients, you're long gone.

Hopefully by now you're beginning to see why someone who goes into conflict intent on only using fists is so easy to beat. He may have a pair of kings, but you have four aces.

More Low-Down, Dirty Tricks

You may think so, but until you have seen two adult males join in combat you have no idea what could be involved. I'll give you a hint—until gang members went wild with guns in the last several years, the ages of 25–35 were the most deadly. Go look it up in the old Uniform Crime Report at your local library.

² Regardless of what the evil sensei in the movies says.

³ I'm talking about the here and now. Many gang members have a fatalistic outlook that one day they won't make it. This combined with a—believe it or not—lack of knowledge that it will hurt when it does come makes them suicidally aggressive. I know of one incident in which a shot gang-banger was lying there screaming "It hurts! It's not supposed to hurt!" They jump when they should back off, which makes them doubly dangerous. Conversely, when things go sideways they are far less able to handle it. It is most definitely a bad news-good news situation.

⁴ And this is why you have to go take your monkey brain to amygdala obedience school. I am going to restress that I highly recommend you go to a bona fide combat course. I know they are expensive, but IMPACT, Model Mugging, Awakening the Warrior Within, Rocky Mountain Combat Applications Training, etc., are all highly recommended. These are not martial artists who run a regular school and then put on a "course." They've spent loads of time, research, and energy putting together something that works, based on scenario/adrenal training.

⁵ Something I teach in my professional use of force classes is that pain and emotion are motivational messages. When you are feeling either of them, you are compelled to react. You HAVE to do something about the message and do it NOW! Notice that nowhere did I say you had to react intelligently, rationally, or logically; all I said is you have to react. Generally, the reaction is based on getting the message to stop, not fixing what is causing the message. This small difference can result in wildly different reactions. Let's say you're the boss on a loading dock and you have an employee who's messing up. When you tell him that he's about to get fired for his behavior, he gets angry. Instead of improving his performance (which would be solving the problem), he reacts

by thinking you are picking on him. Not only is he totally ignoring what he did to cause the situation, he is focusing on his emotional message. The easiest way to stop the message is to stop you. Are we seeing a target being painted on our chests yet? Hope so, because people trying to stop the message rather than solving the problem are the cause for much violence.

6   There is an old Chinese martial arts story about three competing archers. At a great distance, they shoot at the target that—for some obscure reason—is a fish. All the arrows hit the fish's head. It looks like a tie. When they ask the first archer what he was shooting at he says, "The fish." The second says "The fish's head." The third says, "The fish's eye." He won. You're only as accurate as you practice to be, which is why you should always aim at the fish's eye in practice.

7   In this situation, drawing the bow can either be used to draw the guy's arm out to create a direct line to his body weight, or allow you to get a better grip (say one hand on the shoulder, the other at the elbow). In either case, when you have him where you want him, lock down and throw your body weight into it with the pivot.

8   I know of only one person who has died from such an impact. He was a cowboy whose belt got hooked on the saddlehorn when his horse reared. He leaned forward as the horse's head whipped back. The reason the cribriform plate (the horizontal section of skull behind the nasal cavity) broke loose and was driven into his brain is that the rest of his face was shattered, too. Your fist is not as massive as a horse's head. It's not likely that you can hit hard enough to crush someone's skull without a tool.

9   Combine it with an Alien face grab, a quick whirl around the horizontal axis, and Bob's your uncle. Of course, he's going to be in a world of hurt.

10   If you're on a tight budget, aside from the used-sports equipment places, you can often find cheap heavy bags at garage and yard sales. Not long ago, I scored a 60-pound bag for four dollars. Thrift shops occasionally get them in too. Make it a habit to swing by now and then.

[11]   I have a teaching maxim, which is, "Don't attack the man; attack his systems." If he can't walk, breathe, see, or stay upright, he's not much of a threat.

Manly Man Behavior

*You can't govern by sitting in your studies
and thinking how good you are. You've got
to fight for all you know how, and you'll find
a lot of able men willing to fight you.*
—Theodore Roosevelt

When he was a young man, my grandfather
worked the high iron. He riveted steel I-beams
together on buildings way above ground level. One
day he had what is now called a "workplace accident" (back then they called it an "oops"). A board
he was standing on gave way and he fell. This was-
n't a straight fall, though—on each floor underneath
him were plywood sheets. When he'd hit, each
board would stop him for a moment before giving
way. He fell 13 stories, one story at a time, with
major impacts every step of the way.

When he finally hit the ground, the foreman
came up to him as he was lying there in shock and
asked, "Anything broken?"

When my grandfather replied no, the foreman
said, "OK, get back up there." Grandpa dusted himself off and went back to work.

Now I want you to consider the hardest punch that you've ever thrown in a sparring match and ask yourself if that one punch would stop someone who could get up from a 13-story fall and go back to work?

Such people are out there, and most of them work in professions where physical stress and trauma are just part of their jobs; e.g., construction workers, ranchers, heavy equipment operators, roughnecks, manual laborers, etc. They take more bumps, lumps, and thumps during a normal work week than you take in a full-contact match.

In my professional life, I have ridden collapsing buildings to the ground; been blown up; been slammed in the head by beams; fallen from roofs; had 55-gallon drums slam me into walls; been stepped on; and moved, hauled, and thrown tons upon tons of dirt, rocks, steel, iron, wood, and everything in-between. And that was just one type of work. In my other professions I've been punched, kicked, kneed, elbowed, slammed into walls, head-butted, whacked by pool cues, slammed into and onto cars, and crashed through doors. That's professional. What I do for the in-laws these days gets me kicked, bit, stepped on, and bodychecked into fences by 1,500 pounds of soon-to-be-Big-Macs.[1] What do you think a roundhouse kick is going to do to me? It may be the best one you've ever thrown in your life, but I've had worse and kept on going.

I'm not the only gorilla in my family tree. My grandfather not only worked the high iron, but worked in a mine, roughnecked it, and had a whole host of other physically brutal jobs. That was one tough hombre. Want to take a shot at my 6-foot-2-inch loading-dock-working biker brother? Doing 90 mph on his motorcycle, he gets hit harder by bugs than most blows thrown in full-contact tournaments.

While it may sound like I'm pounding my chest, realize my family was NOT the toughest in my old neighborhood! There were folks out there who could dribble us like basketballs. There are entire families out there that are human fire ants.[2] You can pound on them for 30 minutes and all you do is manage to piss them off.

Hopefully, you can begin to see why I get so frustrated by the "I'm invincible" attitude that many sports martial artists have. Martial artists are NOT the only people out there who know how to fight. They're not the only people who can take a punch and keep on coming. Furthermore, there are lots people who can, and HAVE, survived in real-life "no rules" contests.

The reason I'm telling you this is to point out three major flaws in what many martial artists call self-defense training. I want you to consider these points very carefully because they define a major difference between training for self-defense and any other martial arts focus.

FLAWS IN MARTIAL ARTS "SELF-DEFENSE" TRAINING

Most martial artists train to fight a lesser opponent

They train as if everyone they fight will be weaker, less trained, or less physically competent. In many cases, martial arts training isn't an unbeatable advantage; it's just sort of an equalizer if you have to go up against a construction worker. It's his greater strength, constitution, and commitment to hurt you vs. your training. Figure the least you're going to be fighting is someone who's bigger and stronger.

Ninety percent of the trouble is caused by 10 percent of the people

Don't train to fight the 90 percent of the population that is harmless. If your goal is to learn self-defense, assume that you're going to be fighting a member of that 10 percent. While most of those who pick fights are punks or bullies (or fools who think they are invincible), there are some hard-core, dangerous people out there. They know just as much, if not more about fighting and hurting people than you do! (And he's a construction worker to boot!)

If the guy wasn't sure he could take you, he wouldn't have moved against you in the first place

This one seems to elude most martial artists. But it harkens back to the "uh-oh" feeling you should have when you tell the guy you're a black belt and he doesn't back off. The most common response I hear from martial artists is "Well, he doesn't know what I can do." OK, granted, maybe the guy has seriously underestimated you and your abilities. He could be wrong about being able to take you.

On the other hand, you don't know what he can do either! Or what he has up his sleeve! He could just as likely be *right* about his ability to take you! Assume the reason he's attacking is that he knows something you don't. That means he's taken your measure and decided that he can get away with attacking you! One of the things he might have considered already IS that you are a martial artist! This had better be a sobering thought.

In conclusion on this particular thread, I want you to assume that the minimum you will be fighting is a construction worker, and train accordingly. What does that mean?

1) Practice hitting hard. Go out and pound the

heavy bag. Then get a friend suited up in protective gear and pummel him. Learn how to throw powerful, fast, and effective blows!

2) Learn how to keep on attacking. Chain your attacks. Keep them coming. If the guy can take 13 punches, you throw 14! (I know I said it should end in three, but I'm trying to make a point here.)

3) Learn to attack coming and going. No wasted motion. If you pull back, make it an attack— bring something tender along with you.

4) Learn targeting. The human body is constructed in such a way that a strike to the right point will cause major trauma, but the same blow three inches off is useless. Know where to strike!

5) Learn to use your fear! Don't fight it! Fear is one of your greatest allies. If you learn how to channel it, you can use it to defeat your foe instead of letting it defeat you. Most fights aren't lost because of skill or strength, most fights are lost because of fear.

6) Realize that the person who attacks you is experienced in getting his way through violence. He'll jump into violence faster than you can imagine because he's learned he can succeed. From this experience, however, most people get sloppy. Nine times out of 10 they rely more on bad attitude, their ability to take a shot or two, and the unexpectedness of their attack to win. This, more than any actual fighting skill, is what you will be facing most often. Don't give him a chance to figure out what went wrong with his plan.

7) Of anything that is presented as "self-defense," ask yourself, "Would that work against a stronger/bigger opponent?" If you're not sure, try to resist as your partner clamps down on you. If you can't effectively control a training

partner who isn't cooperating, you definitely won't be able to do it against some knuckledragger who is out to hurt you. Doing this winnows out much of the chaff that has crept into the martial arts on this subject. I'm also talking about what you can comfortably do. Many techniques are actually "size relevant." What works for a small man doesn't always work for a large one and vice versa.

8) Assume there will be a weapon involved. Tailor your defenses to not being touched. That means paying lots of attention to footwork and getting off the line of an attack. Aim your blocks in as deeply as you can to avoid the weapon in an attacker's hand. And practice ending it as fast as you can.

9) Practice Fluffy! Get with a partner who is fully geared up and see exactly how good he is at keeping you from getting to the door when you really want to go there. Either that or you get padded up and see how easy it is to keep someone from crawling over you.

10) Train against dynamic attacks. Nobody will just grab and stand there like they show in the martial arts rags. Momentum will always be integral to real attacks. For example, a grab/bear hug from behind will either be a tackle, a backward pull, or a lift. Which one it is will dramatically affect what you need to do. Also train for a punch to follow any grab. That's reality.

You don't have to do these all the time. Stay with your particular focus—it's a good thing. But when you step into this focus, realize that it's not a warm, fuzzy place. Train for reality, not what you think is the actual problem. That means training to handle tough, dangerous opponents who want to hurt you.

Get someone fully padded up and protected. Chest gear, head and eye gear, shin and forearm protection, everything . . . get that guy in FULL armour. Then proceed to crawl all over him. Hit him with everything you've got, again and again, until he goes down.

It takes a certain ruthlessness to strike a fellow human being with full force. Most people won't do it unless they are enraged. Unfortunately, you seldom reach the point of rage at the same time as your attacker. You have to learn to attack with full consciousness of what it is that you are doing. You have made a rational decision to hurt someone to prevent them from hurting you. By actually attacking an armoured human being you will learn A LOT about the realities of fighting. Stuff that until you've actually been there, you cannot imagine.

I strongly recommend you do all of these exercises at your school under an instructor's supervision instead of in your backyard with a friend. These things tend to get wild, and people get hurt if they're not done with the proper safety precautions.

Do role playing where some guy screams, howls, barks, and drools in your face before attacking. Train your amygdala through experience. Without the I-know-I-can-handle-this-because-I've-done-it-before deep memory, you're likely to freeze like a kid with his hand in cookie jar when confronted by this emotional energy. With such training you can look at such a person and say, "Get off mah land," and he'll know you're quite capable of backing it up.

Finally, I will harp on it again: Go out and take a combat course from an established institution like IMPACT, Model Mugging, or any other group I mentioned. There's a list of them in the back of the book. I've seen a lot of knock-offs, and martial arts schools try to run their own. I'll tell you the truth:

Many of these scare me. There is *so* much stuff that goes on in people's brains with this kind of training that it is critical to go to professionals. Until you've actually been there, you have no idea what combat can do to your head. These programs have been developed over the years to handle the deep psychological issues that arise from awakening this part of the human psyche. The idea is to avoid post traumatic stress disorder, not create it.

These are just a few things you can do to make your martial arts street effective. But perhaps the best thing is to look at what you can do to avoid getting into conflict in the first place. There have been many times in life when getting up in someone's face got my butt kicked. And there have been many times when someone who thought he could get away with crowding me discovered exactly how wrong he was. Over the years I have learned the value of avoiding conflict because I learned the cost of conflict. Perhaps one of the most important things I ever heard on this subject was from the unknown man who said, "Don't fight unless there is something worth winning."

Fighting costs. Win, lose, or draw, there will be a price tag attached. When you realize that victory isn't guaranteed, you begin to see that the price might just be higher than you want to pay. This tends to make you cautious about jumping into battle without good reason.

A key trick to survival in this world is learning how to recognize the pathways that lead to conflict. The best way not to end up there is not to get onto the road at all. That doesn't just mean what would lead to conflict where you're from, but what would cause conflict elsewhere.

Recently, my sweetie Dianna and I were watching a program about the Donner Party.[3] It mentioned how a fight broke out between two men in the wagon train when one tried to pass the other. In the resulting argument, one of the men pulled a knife and stabbed the other, killing him.

Dianna was shocked that something so insignificant could lead to a killing. I looked at her and said, "It happens all the time." From my past, I couldn't understand her not understanding how such a thing could happen. That's the difference in upbringing. Where she is from such things don't happen. Where I'm from people do it all the time. It all depends on what you're used to as to whether or not you expect it. Problem is you never know where the other guy is coming from.

I'll give you a free hint: It's not what the argument is about that causes the killing. That, most often, is just the excuse. Those two men had been locking horns for weeks prior—a covered wagon race was the just the catalyst for what they already wanted to do. In a roundabout way, the same thing applies to the stray idiot who jumps in your face for no reason. He already has something eating him. He's just looking for an excuse to take it out on the world, and he happened to choose you.

This kind of idiot is easy to step wide of. There's nothing in it for you to fight such a clown. Yet every day, thousands of people are dragged into fights by these kinds of jokers. Some bozo who's looking for a target gives you a hard look or a rude word, and you fire the same back. Bang! Next thing you know you're in the middle of it. Thing is, when he walked in the door he was prepared to take it to extremes. Were you expecting to go that far when you took the bait? Probably not. That's why these clowns usually win. If someone throws the bait out, look carefully before you react.

Remember how I said earlier that the times for

violence seldom involve anger on your part? Actually, I think I said seldom involve strong emotion, but anger is a biggie in most fights. This especially applies to the problem that is working its way toward boiling over. If you have problems with someone it's generally better to try to negotiate them out. If that doesn't work, just keep away from each other. When you're both involved and pissed, it's way too easy to go over the line.

The root of this problem is most people don't know the difference between being assertive and being aggressive. Go out and pick up a few books on the subject and you'll begin to see that there is a big difference.

The problem about not knowing the difference is that assertiveness stops most situations from escalating to violence, while aggressiveness almost always guarantees it goes there. Thing is, you might not be in control when it blows. I've seen a lot of people get slammed into walls over the years. A significant majority of them had shocked expressions on their faces when it happened. It wasn't the pain that caused that expression, although that was part of it. Rather, it was more that the snide, vicious, or rude comment they had just made hadn't resulted in the other person limping off in defeat. Instead, the other person was starting to jackhammer their face into mush.

Take a trip to the nearest unabridged dictionary and look up the word "violence." Using one of the Random House definitions, it is "rough or immoderate vehemence, as of feeling or language." Violence doesn't have to be physical. In fact, some of the most violent people have never thrown a punch in their lives. Their weapons are words.

Well, bad news here folks, violence attracts violence. It doesn't matter if you think you are being violent or not. What you put out comes back. The hair-ball of it all is that what you put out may not be the same type that comes back. You throw words and he throws fists back. How do you think fights start?

The reason I highly recommend you go out and read up on the difference between being assertive and aggressive is simple. Most people, when they think they are just defending themselves, are in fact attacking. The comment you think will convince the guy to back off could in truth be the very thing that sets him off.

This situation is way more slippery than most people imagine. When you are reacting emotionally, you are reacting to internal messages, not external ones. That makes it hard to judge when those lines have been crossed. I have seen many otherwise intelligent, rational people turn into complete were-wolves when their feelings were hurt or when they felt threatened or insulted. The thing about it is, they have no idea how they appear to others, much less the effect they are having.

Years ago, I had a great many people come up to me and say they had seen me in a movie. (Well, not exactly me, but someone they thought had been modeled after me.) The movie was *Full Metal Jacket*. They kept on saying that there was one line in particular that reminded them of me. After about a dozen people had said this, I thought I should go see what they were talking about. The character they were talking about was named "Animal Mother." OK, well, we had part of something in common. When I saw the movie all I could think of was, "What an asshole!"

The real slap in the face was the one line that they thought was so much me. In the scene, the squad is standing around the bodies of fallen com-rades, and each is saying something over them.

Animal Mother's comment is, "Better you than me."

In the middle of my indignation, it hit me. I HAD said that! And in exactly those circumstances! I knew why I had said it, and I felt perfectly justified at the moment. (I didn't like the guy anyway.) But all of a sudden, I was faced with what I looked like to other people. It was not a pleasant experience. It was, however, one of the things that started me turning around and coming out of the streets.

The reason I told you this story is to let you know how easy it is to not only to lose sight of how we appear to others, but to lose sight of the significance of our own actions. Even though I felt justified in what I said about the dead guy, it was a rude, barbarous, and horrible thing. In all honesty, if someone who'd held that person dear had heard me say that, he would have been justified in flying across the table to try and kick my ass. I probably would have sat there later and said, "I was just minding my own business when all of a sudden this jerk went off on me!" That's not accepting responsibility for the fact I had said something that, had I heard it about one of my fallen friends, would have sent me off, too. See, I could say it but others couldn't. Yeah, that's a reasonable standard. Ppppffffftttt!

There is a saying in Proverbs: Do unto others as you would have them do unto you. There's something slippery about the phrasing. To me it always sounded a little, "Gee, it would be nice," but it never conveyed a sense of immediacy. It wasn't until I was reading the original Jewish version that I got the, "Oh, is that what they mean?" reaction. It was a little more clear: Do unto others as will be done unto you. Well whaddaya know, they knew about karma too. Or for those of you of a less esoteric bent, payback is a bitch.

Looking back, I now wonder how many of the

fights I got into weren't just some guy coming out of nowhere like it seemed at the time. I wondered how many of them were because of something I said or did that stepped on other people's toes. Exactly how closely did I resemble that guy Animal Mother, who said and did whatever was on his mind with no regard to the consequences or how it affected others? If that was the case, no wonder I was always in the middle of it.

Before you just assume that trouble seeks you out, take a look at how you are coming across to others. This is a major part of knowing how to avoid going down the road to conflict. Words are weapons: Know this before you speak. Watch for this behavior and you will see how often people lash out verbally. For whatever reason, they feel perfectly justified in doing it, often without realizing exactly what it is that they are doing. Or, worse, they don't realize how easy it is for the situation to escalate past just hurtful words—especially when they are dealing with someone from a different background than theirs. People who use words as weapons often don't realize there are areas where blood is the price for such behavior. And if you're not willing to back it up physically, don't say it.

Knowing that there is a price tag attached to conflict is one of the best reasons for learning how to avoid it. This is especially true if you regularly deal with other socioeconomic levels or people from other cultures. Often this includes dealing with fire ants. Over the years, I have seen many people do things that are perfectly acceptable where they are from, yet it's something that makes a fire ant stand up.

Not too long ago, I heard about a world famous martial artist who made the mistake of picking a fight in a bar in Oregon. It was a local lumberjack bar out in the sticks, so we can assume his presence there was no accident. The logger who picked him up and used him as a pool cue didn't care that this guy was a master of obscure and dangerous arts and had a reputation in the martial arts community for being a real fire-eater. Bubba just don't take kindly to that kind of behavior in his waterin' hole.

Now, I'm not saying that you're going to do what that moron did and go a thousand miles out of your way to pick a fight with a lumberjack just to prove your fighting skills. But I want you think of some ways by which you might find yourself in an altercation with a human fire ant. The guy you cut off in traffic and who gets out of his car at the next stoplight could be one. The guy your girlfriend/wife decides to give a piece of her mind to could be one. Even if you don't travel between social levels, there are many ways that you can get into conflict with such people.

What's worse is if you go around thinking that your martial arts make you a stud. You set up a red flag for bullies, brawlers, and tough guys to come up and pick a fight with you. I hate to tell you, but this happens even if you're doing it just to keep the tough guys from bothering you. You may convince the 90 percent to walk wide of you, but that 10 percent is still going to be drawn to you like flies. The real problem with this kind of behavior is that you might accidentally step on a fire ant's toes. To the casual glance, fire ants look like the very thing you're trying to shoo away. Free hint: If there's a tough guy over in the corner minding his own business, leave him alone. Don't set about to show him how tough you are.

Not long ago Dianna and Tony J. dragged me kicking and screaming to an international tournament. We decided that the best place to be was up in the balcony. Not only for a better view, but to keep out of the hazy cloud of testosterone that hung over the floor. I ain't never seen so many puffed-up, arms-thrown-back studs in my life. With the amount of attitude floating around, I was amazed that there weren't any obvious problems. This especially in light of the fact that they hadn't metal detected us at the door like they used to back home.[4] When I saw how the competitors fought I realized where all that attitude was coming from. Apparently the style's idea of strategy was to let your opponent shin kick you in the thigh until you won when he suffered a heart attack from the exertion. This old fart decided right then and there this was most definitely a young man's game.

I'm going to go out on thin ice here and point something out. Many sports-oriented martial artists are big fish in little ponds. They don't spend any time out on construction sites, in biker bars, or in rough neighborhoods and they don't get tough-guy manners. Yes, believe it or not, there is "street etiquette." The purpose of manners is so people don't have to kill each other.

The best summation I ever heard about manners is from Robert A. Heinlein: "Etiquette is the oil that the machinery of society runs on." This oil becomes real important when you are surrounded by people who can inflict major damage. Think about it: A room full of armed men is much more polite than a room where only one person is armed. Believe it or not, I have seen better manners in biker bars than I have in fine restaurants. A good rule of thumb is to assume everyone you deal with is either armed or as good a fighter as you. It's amazing how fast you'll get manners.

This is especially true if you are in a school where the focus is sport competition. When you're nervous about the dangers you might face on the street, I know how easy it is to see these schools as the answer. I know the competition fighters and instructors look like real fire eaters, but if you pick up that attitude, you're going to call down more grief than you will avoid. This is especially true if you are in a situation where you regularly have to deal with the real thing: work, school, neighborhood, etc.

Two young guys who want to show each other how tough they are will huff, puff, and ruffle their feathers. Crusty looks fly around the room thicker than moths near a nightlight. Voices get loud, postures get exaggerated, and all sorts of other stuff happens to let the other guy know who's tougher. If this display doesn't work they often end up in a fight.

It is the sign of an inexperienced punk that he has to come up and get in someone's face or show everyone that he's the baddest dude in the room. What I'm about to say will do more for keeping you out of fights than most anything else: Real tough guys know that "when two tigers fight, one dies; the other is wounded." Because of this, they really don't want to mix it up for no reason. They're not looking for trouble because they know its cost. But if it is unavoidable, they are willing to pay the price to win.

Here's an interesting thing to observe. When two heavy hitters are in the same area, they handle it one of two ways. One, they make friends with each other. That's right, they become buddies and avoid conflict altogether. I'm cool, you're cool, it's cool. Let's relax. The other way? They ignore each other. As long as each stays out of the other's way there is no problem. "You got your side of the room, I got mine." This means not throwing crusties or staring at the guy. Don't get loud. Don't do anything that attracts the guy's attention AND expect the same in return. You simply attend to your business and your friends. And let him attend to his.

This is the difference between troublemakers and fire ants. A fire ant will let you have your side if you let him have his. The troublemaker, however, will insist on bringing it to you. Good news though, *Roadhouse* had it right: "Those who come looking for trouble really aren't that good at it." They think they are, but if attitude was all it took, we'd all be famous.

When you find yourself in an area with someone who looks like a piece of bad-assed real estate, keep a watch on him out of the corner of your eye and go about what you're doing. If you're with someone, tell him or her to warn you if they see the guy coming over toward you. My personal favorite is to sit with my side to him or with my back toward him (with a mirror in front of me, of course). That way I can pay attention to the people I'm with and avoid having to respond to any crusties he's throwing my way.

There is a neat thing about all of this. If the guy starts maddogging you and you're not taking the bait, most times he convinces himself that you're scared of him and settles back with what a stud he is. When that happens he most often leaves you alone. It's amazing how much trouble you can avoid by just going about your business.

If the guy starts getting boisterous or obnoxious to get your attention, leave the area. He's a trouble-maker looking to prove something. There's nothing to be gained by locking horns. Learning to walk away from fights where there is nothing to win is the biggest sign of being a pro.

If the guy confronts you, keep in mind your only goal is to end it as fast as possible and get out of there. Not to win, not to prove how tough you are.

Stud muffins is going to be in for a real big surprise if he tries anything.

Sun Tzu said the greatest victories are achieved without a blow ever being struck. A fight avoided is the greatest victory. If you are thinking you have to be rough, tough, and show everyone how much of a manly man you are by not leaving, that's complete nonsense. Nobody else in that room is going to know what you're thinking. They're not looking at it like you are. They don't see a loss of face by not tangling with a troublemaker. To them that's common sense, not cowardice. The only thing jumping up and being a manly man will get you is hurt. Even if you win, you're going to have pain. And for what? You think you've proved you're not a coward, but everyone else thinks you're an idiot.

If you have this idea that you're not supposed to back down because you're a martial artist, reconsider it. Become a professional. What's to be gained by fighting? If the profit doesn't exceed the pain, don't do it.

It's not just you and him that fighting affects, but everyone else in the room. It's going to affect their opinion of you, as well. It's a thin line you walk here. Public opinion is a fickle thing. In the eyes of others it's easy to go from someone who is trying to protect himself into being a bigger monster than the guy who started it.

Staying there and applying a few hits too many will make you the aggressor, both in the eyes of the observers and the law. Being seen trying to escape, i.e., taking the Fluffy attitude, will save you if the police are called in. You didn't stand there and beat on him, you split. You didn't want to fight him in the first place and when it happened the only thing you wanted to do was get out of there. Yeah, he got hurt, but it happened as you were trying to escape when he attacked you. When the police show up and start asking questions, people remember this, and that's what they tell the police. This can go a long way toward keeping you from being arrested. Your statement and actions are all consistent.

There is another REALLY good reason for leaving. A fight doesn't end when you knock someone down. You also have to deal with the guy when he gets up. A real common reaction of that 10 percent who are the troublemakers is to get up, go out, and get a tool. They now know that they can't take you head-on, so they get help. Whether that means with a gun, knife, or friends, they come back looking for you. That's why you don't want to be there. This also applies to people you got to back down without using physical force.

If you still think you want to stick around after a ruckus, consider this: Everyone who has been around has stories about shotgun blasts through the window, drive-bys, ambushes in the parking lots, wild chases through the streets, and sometimes bodies hitting the ground. All of these stories come from not leaving an area immediately after an altercation. Nobody is immune to a shotgun blast from the shadows, folks, and that happens.

If you do get in a conflict with someone, lay low for a few weeks and watch to make sure he doesn't back up on you. It's a sure bet that the guy will be looking for you. Don't go right back to the place where you had the problem. If he can find a way to sneak up on you and nail you when you're not paying attention, he'll do it. Don't make it easy for him by hanging out in the place where you and he mixed it up. Let it defuse.

Even then, you still might have bought yourself a feud by fighting the guy. I'm Scottish. Knowledge of the feud was fed to me with my mother's milk, but for most people it's a surprise. It does exist. The guy who HAS to win, will keep coming at you until he does. Not only that, but certain cultures (the street included) insist on it. Ever notice how many proverbs about revenge the Italians have? That should tell you something. What do you think a gang war is? These are just a few examples: It's out there.

I've been in feuds that only ended when I moved away. Every time they couldn't take me out it was an affront to the group's honor and they kept coming. Always assume that you're not fighting one guy, but his friends and family. If he's got lots of both, they can keep coming long after you're tired of the whole affair.

There are a lot more idiots and troublemakers out there than criminals, psychos, and rapists. You'll run into them more than you will the latter. Unfortunately, dealing with them is more of a gray area than with criminals. In a sense, a mugger or jump-out-of-the bushes rapist is easier to deal with because you know where they stand. Who knows which way a froggy troublemaker is going to jump? Or what trouble he'll cause you afterward. Bright boy wasn't smart enough to figure out that he shouldn't mess with you in the first place, so who knows what other rocket scientist decisions he'll make?

All in all, when it comes to dealing with troublemakers, stay low, keep moving, and choose your battles carefully.

---

[1] To say nothing about getting my butt paddled by a saddle when the cowboys decide to trot a few miles. In case you're wondering what this city boy is doing herding cattle in the boonies of the West, the answer is, saying, "We don't have this problem where I'm from . . ." a WHOLE lot! This "Boyz inna'choya" routine is a definite change of pace. We won't

even talk about having to do it all in the middle of a blizzard. But at least I now know the difference between a cow and a heifer . . . I think.

2 For those of you who don't have fire ants where you are from, let me give you an idea of how tough they are: As a kid I once spent about 30 minutes trying to kill one of these little S.O.B.s. I stomped it, I jumped on it, I dropped rocks on it, but the thing just wouldn't lay down and die. It was dead, it just refused to act like it. Years later, when I saw one in my house, I went after it with a knife. Dianna (who comes from a place where they don't have the little buggers) thought I was overreacting taking a knife to an ant. That is, until a friend told her he would have used a .38. They are tough little boogers.

3 One of the first recorded cases of cannibalism in the United States. A wagon train without an experienced wagonmaster, doing about eight other levels of stupidity, tried to cross the mountains with winter coming on. They ended up snowed in and having to eat each other. Amazingly enough, it was the guy they kicked out for the killing that ended up saving most of them.

4 I hadn't been to a tourney since the riot at the Muay Thai fights prompted my ex to put her foot down about attending such events. Something about flying chairs bothered her for some reason.

Afterword

In my life I've been in more scrapes, jams, fights, and furballs than any intelligent person should ever have been in. If there are those who question my intelligence for having done some of the stupid and dangerous things that I did in my past, all I have to say is "You're right." I'm the first to say add my name to the list that says, "That was real stupid." While it qualified me to write this and my other books about the realities of violence in the street, it also cost me a whole lot of blood, pain, and hassles throughout my life.

Violence is not a game. Nor is it something you want to engage in frivolously or via a whim de jour. Unfortunately, there are many people in this world who don't hold to these opinions. Such folks can and will make your life miserable. They have no compunction about bringing violence into your life to get what they want. These people can show up in your life at any time and anywhere. The damage they can cause can last a lifetime—that's if the rest of your life isn't 30 seconds long.

However, having said this, I'd also like to say that dedicating your life to preparing for a fight that might not ever happen is a great way to miss out on living. There is much more to life than fighting. If you allow your fear of not being good enough to win that mythological ultimate fight to drive you, to consume your every waking moment, to push everything else out of your awareness—well, you're not going to have a good time in this life.

The truth is, you don't have to be the best; all you have to be is good enough.

I never knew this growing up. In real life there aren't blue ribbons saying "You're the best that's ever been"; there's just handling what life throws you. No blue ribbons and no thunderous applause, but there is a great deal of self-respect. When you can consistently function to the best of your abilities, then you'll realize "Good enough is pretty damned good."

Whether or not you're good enough doesn't come from the outside, it comes from the inside. A friend of mine once told me how to counter skeptics who say, "Well, you can't prove it." Instead of trying to prove it to them (an impossible job), ask them, "What would you accept as proof?" This puts the burden of defining what is "proof" back onto them. Then these people who will always find fault can't endlessly raise the ceiling of proof.

The reason I mention this is that we sometimes do this to ourselves. Many of us have an idea of what it means to be "the best," and every time we get close to that, *ZIP*—up go the standards. With me, the way I used to do it was with fear. I believed that a tough guy wasn't afraid. I'd seen all the movies about he-men with grim, stony looks on their faces who'd knock the snot out of hundreds of opponents. More importantly, I saw the tough guys in my neighborhood with total hard-core confidence running roughshod over everyone. Those guys scared me. Deep down I was terrified that I wasn't good enough to stop them from hurting me.

I was different, I was weird, I was small, and I felt like I had a target painted on my chest. No matter what I did, I'd keep on running into them. Well, I'm also what is called counterphobic, which means if something scares me I attack it. I threw myself into the very lifestyle that scared me. Instead of doing everything I could to steer clear from these guys, I would go to the places where we WOULD cross paths. I ended up locking horns with them at every turn. Every time I had a run-in with them I was freaking out. I truly believed that a manly man wasn't supposed to be afraid. The fact that I was afraid when we jammed meant that I wasn't a he-man.

Every time I felt fear I threw myself further and further into both training and the lifestyle where I'd run into these clowns. I went into hard-core training. I'd beat on trees and steel girders, get pounded by training partners, learn every weapon I possibly could and then spar with real weapons, grind cigarettes out on my knuckles, and have people whomp on me so I could learn how to take a punch and keep on going. I trained for what I thought was out there. Then I'd go out into the streets of Los Angeles and look for tough guys to test myself against. I would actively throw myself into situations where I would end up mixing it up with the guys who scared me. Every time I did this and found myself scared, I'd dive back into training even harder.

What I didn't realize was what it looked like from the outside. I developed a reputation for being a real fire-eater. People would look at me and say, "Whoa, that dude can take care of himself." But, because I got scared every time I got into a situation, the only thing that was proven to me was that I was faking it. I wasn't there yet. It didn't matter how extreme it got, people shooting at me, knives, chains, car jacks, multiple opponents, guerrilla warfare . . . the situations kept on getting hairier and hairier. And I kept on diving back into it again and again, trying to defeat my fear.

See, from where I was looking at it, the situation hadn't changed. What I didn't see was those people who had terrified me earlier were now stepping way wide of me. Those guys I had thought were so big and bad were, in fact, really small time in the scheme of things. But instead of relaxing with what I could do, I was still afraid. I kept on focusing on guys who would scare me. I kept on looking for rougher and tougher. Every time I faced one of them down, I'd unconsciously raise the ceiling again. I'd look around and find a bigger, badder, meaner boogeyman that I could affix my fear to. I kept on jumping farther and farther into it trying to find the place where I wasn't afraid anymore.

There finally came a day when the Universe back-handed me with the gentle message of "Hey Stupid, wake up and smell the coffee!" I looked around and realized that the standard of proof I had been demanding of myself wasn't true. I realized that I was sitting among those considered the best of the best. I'd gotten to the top of the pyramid and you know what they all freely admitted? Being scared!

There's a good reason for being scared—THIS STUFF IS DANGEROUS!!! They knew it. They admitted it, and they knew they weren't invincible. They lived with their mortality. Each of them knew that if they screwed up it would cost them their lives. They lived with it every day. And they all used their fear! They didn't let it drive them into obsessiveness, but they used it to hone their skills, to keep them aware and alert. They made it a servant, not the master of their lives. They lived with their mortality rather than denying it or controlling it. That is what gave them the edge, and it was that edge—not being "invincible"—that made them the best.

I began to look back over my life and realize what I had done. I had, indeed, been in hairy situations. Situations that scared the bejeebers out of me. I'd handled them and come out intact. What I hadn't done was handle my fear. I could jackslap a gang member with no problem, I could survive being hunted by entire gangs, I could back down a biker with just a glance, but what I couldn't do was accept that I was good enough. The boogeyman in my head was who I was really afraid of. I kept projecting him onto others. I kept trying to find him out there and beat him up.

I finally realized I'd fought him and beaten him a thousand times, but I'd never defeated him. Every time I'd win a fight, he'd go away and come back to haunt me on another's face. I finally managed to defeat him. It's funny, the final battle wasn't a fight at all. It was accepting that the boogeyman wasn't out there in the legions of thugs, criminals, and psychos, but within me. I had to realize that I was "good enough." I could handle myself.

The odd thing was that when I realized all of this, I also realized that fear had tried to rob me of living. If you have that same boogeyman, know that he's trying to rob you, too. He's an insidious little bastard that keeps you looking where he wants you to. When I realized that was good enough, I could relax and enjoy life for the first time. I could begin to see the good in life, instead of just the bad, harmful, hateful, and mean.

It was at this time I learned about the four focuses of the martial arts. That's when I began to see the benefits of the different focuses. I've begun to work with them more and more to see where they lead. In closing, my advice to you is not to let fear blind you to the other three focuses. Know this focus to whatever level you need for your lifestyle, but don't dwell on it. You miss a whole lot of good stuff out there if you do. I speak from experience. Don't let fear of violence blind you to everything else. There is a lot of good in this world if you are willing to look.

APPENDIX A

What You're Up Against

---

*You better hope and pray that you're going
to awake back in your own world.*

Shakespeare's Sister
"Stay"

What I would like to do here is address my qualifications to write this book and say the things I do about this subject. I know I speak from experience, but unless you have read my other books there is no way you can know what that means.

I am an ex-streetfighter.

That means a very specific thing where I am from, and what it means is not nice.

There is no "If I ever had to use this stuff, I'd . . ." in what I said in this book. The fact that I am still breathing is based on the fact that I HAVE used this stuff in the real thing. In the same breath, however, I will tell you that being a streetfighter is nothing to brag about. I've encountered a whole lot of people who say "Well, my teacher was a streetfighter. What he teaches us would work in the street."

Oh yeah? Before you tell me about streetfighters, go out and read *The Jungle Book* by Rudyard Kipling, with the monkeys jumping up and down chanting, "It's so because we say it's so." This is not to be disrespectful of what you believe, but to tell you in all sincerity to question such a claim. You can say or claim anything; however, just because you say something that doesn't make it true. Give a listen to any lawyer or liberal arts professor and you'll see what I mean.

A lot of martial art instructors claim to be street-fighters. They brag about how their system is street proven. To listen to these people, you'd think they were real hardcore street savages. And to give them credit, they may have been bouncers and even brawlers. Still, that's a totally different league than streetfighters.

Simply stated, most martial arts teachers who claim to have been streetfighters don't have the stink.

There is a certain psychic odor that comes from growing up and living in the streets. It's a rot that comes from constant exposure to violence, death, alcoholism, drug addiction, sociopathic behavior, poverty, sadism, and viciousness. It's reflected in a person's attitudes, speech patterns, personal inter-actions, and how he looks at the world. It's a certain hardening of the spirit that comes from living years with the attitude of "Do unto others before they do unto you." Add to that the chronic paranoia of hav-ing spent years looking over your shoulder, lest someone you have wronged slithers out of the shad-ow you just passed with revenge on his mind.

When I say I was a streetfighter, it means that I was a vicious, self-centered, misbehaving, drunken, stoned thug among other vicious, self-centered, mis-behaving, drunken, stoned thugs. We were the worst kind of savages. Man to man, mano a mano was bull. Numbers and weapons were always used to increase our odds whenever possible. Once you realized the other side could and would shoot back, you did everything in your power to make sure he never got the chance. You always stacked the deck in your favor. You hit first, and you hit hard enough to make sure he didn't get up. You ran as often as you hit, and you hit from behind as often as you could. Anyone who didn't play that way didn't last too long. The blood, the bullets, and the knives were real. In the streets, life and death were determined by whims, intoxicants, and sheer stupidity.

Being, or having been, a streetfighter is nothing to be proud of, much less brag about. Nor is it something that you turn on and off. It's not a job that you go to and come home from. It's a way of life (and often death), and it's constant. It's living with being the hunter and the hunted every day and night. Knowing that the next corner you turn could end your life, you don't swagger boldly around it. You cautiously turn that corner.

It's not aggressiveness or how many people he's beat up that makes a streetfighter—that's just a sadistic brawler. Such people don't last long in the streets. A brawler goes into places, picks a fight, and then leaves the area to go back to a home far away from the trouble he caused. Streetfighting isn't stomping someone and then contemptuously forgetting them like so many bouncers and brawlers do. It's spending two weeks after a conflict watching approaching cars lest a gun barrel comes poking out of a rolled down window. It's dashing wildly through alleys to escape six guys who suddenly jumped out of a car. Of course, having the guy you beat up waiting in the shadows with a baseball bat as you come out of a door is also loads of laughs to deal with. That is what being a streetfighter is about. It's surviving the aftermath of your actions when someone backs up on you on his terms, not yours.

There's a lot of pain and paranoia involved in being a streetfighter that the fakes don't know about. Standing over a friend's grave is a horrible experience. Spending your life always looking over your shoulder doesn't do your social graces any good. Waking up with the cops pounding on the door for what happened last night really compounds the suffering of a hangover. Long nights spent in the emergency room because someone blindsided you with a beer bottle or scrubbing your friend's blood out of your car seat—those are the experiences of a streetfighter. The scars, both physical and psychic, stand out clearly. Trying to impress people by claiming to be one is like trying to impress people by claiming that you're a leper.

Most people I knew in the "Life" are now either dead, in prison, totally burned out courtesy of drugs or booze, or crippled because of a shadow with a shotgun. That's what happens to most "streetfighters." Those few who do manage to escape know about the downside, and that's why they left. Even people who weren't players, but who grew up in lousy neighborhoods and fought their way out, have the stink. It stays with you forever. Someone who thinks going out and picking fights or working a few months as a bouncer in a local watering hole means he's a streetfighter is mistaken.

You can see why such a life would give someone a spiritual stink. I should know—that was how I was raised and that was the environment I operated in while running in the streets of Los Angeles. Even though I left it behind, the residue still remains with me to this day. It's taken me many long, hard years working to improve myself from that state, and I still don't have it down.

Oh, by the way, something I've noticed for you social climbers: One of the more interesting things about "civilized conversation" isn't so much what you talk about, as it is what you DON'T talk about. If a subject is discussed it's reached round about; you don't just blurt it out. That kind of directness is one of the marks of someone coming from the street, not someone with so-called class.

It's knowing this downside of the "life" that is the litmus test for telling ex-streetfighters from wannabes. Basically, you can now see why someone who brags about being a streetfighter isn't one. What's there to impress people with? "Hi! I'm a dysfunctional, intoxicated thug who hurts people unnecessarily . . . what do you do for a living?" Gee, that goes over well at dinner parties.

In the same way that a lot of camp cooks suddenly became snipers when they returned from Vietnam, a whole lot of martial arts instructors became ex-streetfighters when they opened their schools. It's a marketing ploy. It sounds really good. It attracts students, and people who don't know the difference believe them—thinking that streetfighting and aggressive sports training regimes are the same thing. The problem is, it's not true. If you believe such a person in good faith, you are the one who will bleed to discover what he's teaching won't work in the real thing.

How Your Brain Works

The appearance of things to the mind
is the standard of every action to man.

—Epictetus

In his book *Anything Goes*, Loren Christensen
has a story that had me shrieking in terror.[1] Officer
Adams had practiced a gun disarm again and again.
After he disarmed his training partner, he'd hand
back the gun and do it over again. One night, when
unexpectedly confronted, he disarmed the suspect
AND HANDED THE GUN BACK TO THE GUY! He
did exactly as he had been trained.

Fortunately, his less well-trained partner
showed up and shot the bad guy. Of all the stories I
have ever heard about how ingrained training
habits can show up at the wrong time, this has to
be the worst. Notice I didn't say "bad training
habits," but only "ingrained habits." Simply stated,
the way you train is the way you are going to react.
In the kwoon or dojo you develop civilized respect-
ful habits, and they serve a very good purpose. It's

just that when they show up in a real situation they are not only out of place, but likely to get you hurt.

When they hear me talk about the differences between sparring and fighting, most martial artists come up with a response along the lines of, "Well, I could move differently if I wanted to . . ." Sure, and if pigs could fly there'd be pork in the treetops by morning. Are you thinking you can, at a snap of the fingers, override years of deeply embedded training and know exactly what to change? Are you that aware of what is happening in your subconscious? Do you really believe that you could shift gears fast enough to survive someone swinging a baseball bat as he steps out of the shadows?

Before you get bent thinking that I'm negating your years of training, I highly recommend you go out and buy the book *Emotional Intelligence* by Daniel Goleman. This is the easiest explanation available of the work of neuroscientist Joseph LeDoux.[2] LeDoux's theories about a neurological "back alley" and the amygdala are not only ground-breaking, but inadvertently the strongest scientific explanation I have ever found in support of scenario-based stress training. Once you understand the significance of this stuff, it explains why such training is so effective and in the same breath shows you why a 4th-degree black belt would sit down in shock when attacked.

It has a whole lot to do with deep emotional programming, far, far beneath the realm of conscious thought and rational processes. We're talking real monkey brain stuff, here. Yet, it is the very thing that got your ancestors up the tree for millions of years before the lion could invite them out for lunch. Much of this is based on how your amygdala works.

The important news is that it's how your

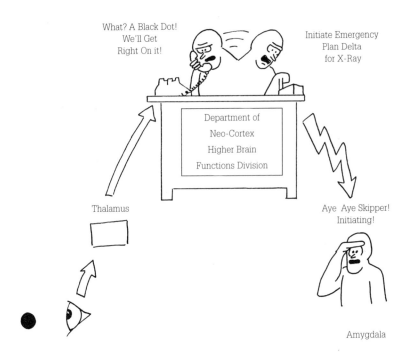

Old neurological model

amygdala is trained—NOT how you are trained—
that will determine the way you will react in a
crisis situation.

It may sound like I just took up glue sniffing to
say that there is a difference between how you and
your monkey brain were trained. But, have faith. It's
easier to understand it if we separate the two.

Looking at them separately makes sense since
the two can give conflicting messages at the same
time. If you say "fight" and it says "flight," you
have problems. Either it's going to win and you will
find yourself beating feet (and later beating yourself
up for being a coward) or you both will lose. While

you're arguing about who is in charge, you're going to get your butt kicked.

This is the old model of how scientists once believed a brain worked. Input came through your eyes, went to the thalamus for translation into brain-speak, and got sent up to your higher brain functions which then decided if it was a threat. If so, the higher brain functions sent the emotionally charged message to react to the amygdala.

The amygdala then dumped adrenaline into your system so you could do whatever that smart old brain of yours told you to do. In other words, you could either fight or run fiercely for survival depending on what was the best choice. This was a nice neat package that put your higher brain functions firmly in charge.

Unfortunately, they scientists were wrong.

Anyone who has been shot at could have told them. But since most scientists have never been shot at, they didn't recognize the flaws of that model. This whole process would take too much time—time you don't have in a real crisis.

See, our nerves fire only so fast. Physiologically speaking, there is a speed limit. Like a trip through the department of motor vehicles, it would take too long for the information to go all the way around with the old model. By that time, either the lion has got you or the shooter has corrected his aim. Bad news, that.

I've seen too many people freeze and react in confusion when confronted by unexpected violence. Fight or flight does not constitute a complicated choice—I've been in situations where I'm still alive because I reacted *without consciously knowing why*! I know when I am thinking, and I know when I'm not. (Boy, did I leave myself open with that statement). What I was doing at that time was not

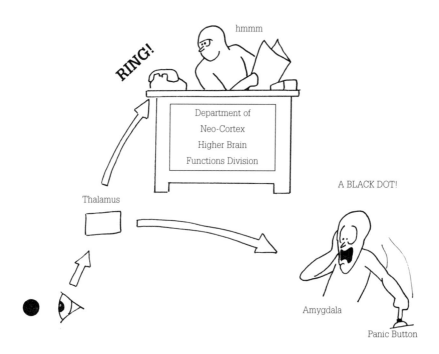

hmmm

RING!

Department of
Neo-Cortex
Higher Brain
Functions Division

A BLACK DOT!

Thalamus

Amygdala

Panic Button

LeDoux's model

rational thought, yet I was reacting! I was not
floundering around going, "Whadda I do? Whadda I
do?" I hear a gunshot, and I suck earth. It's not a
rational reaction; it's an automatic one. This happens way too fast for it to go the long way around.

Let's take a look at what LeDoux found with his
infamous back alley.

The old model explained day to day living. What
it didn't explain was how we react in crisis. When
LeDoux showed up with the back alley theory, it
better explained how we work when things go sideways. It gives us a kind of emergency override system. Here's how it works: the amygdala has a rudi-
mentary set of definitions of what it considers dangerous. The higher brain functions have more
advanced and better structured definitions, but the

amygdala's are pretty basic. In addition to all of this, it has a panic button. Once it slams this panic button you get a strong emotional and adrenaline reaction.

As well as basic definitions and panic buttons, the amygdala has "learned" responses. When it hits the panic button it's got a reaction already lined up. All of a sudden, you're on autopilot doing what the amygdala considers your best reaction.

Where all of this becomes important is that there is a little back alley. While the old model is 95-percent accurate, that other 5 percent is beaucoup importanto. See, the back alley allows for a copy of the incoming messages to be channeled directly to the amygdala. If it sees something it doesn't like, it hits the panic button.

When the amygdala slams that panic button, it tells us to behave in a way that it has learned is the best to handle this situation. Maybe it was a long time ago, but that programming is still there. That is our initial physical and emotional reaction—not what we think!

This is kind of a handy thing to have if you're in a place where hungry lions and tigers and bears have a habit of popping up unexpectedly. When a hungry pussycat comes bounding out from the bushes, an immediate and automatic "RUN!" response is a whole lot better than, "Gee, what are my options at this moment?" Remember the fox and the cat story? Having an automatic fear- and adrenaline-driven "GET UP THE TREE!" response tends to get the job done.

This is not a rational process; it is an emotional and adrenaline-based one. This can work for good or bad. While it can save your life if it's trained properly, if your amygdala takes that same response and hangs it on something minor you can get all sorts of problems. That explains why some people overreact

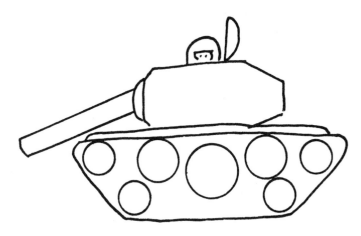

Amygdala in panic

over a small detail. They are absolutely convinced they are engaging in a perfectly appropriate reaction when, in fact, they are bouncing off the walls. Their amygdala has hijacked them.

What is important to recognize is that much of what the amygdala reacts to is emotional input. It not only sees the actions, but it sees the attached emotions. A large part of what it considers danger is strong emotional behavior.

It doesn't matter how long ago it learned it either. When confronted with such a situation again, the amygdala will react as it did before. Ready for a shock? It can easily be said that most fights are lost on an emotional level.

Huh, you say? Bear with me for a moment. Let me point out that most people who train in the martial arts do so in a pleasant environment. While you may have lots of experience with people throwing punches at you, how much experience do you have with people attacking you in unbridled anger?

I mean howling, screaming, gonna rip your head

off and piss down the hole anger? How about if it just came out of nowhere? There you are one minute minding your own business and the next thing you know some red-eyed werewolf is launching at you. Let's just assume this is a little outside your normal daily activities.

Let us further assume that this kind of thing doesn't happen too often in your dojang. So where are you going to learn how to handle it?

AH HA! The amygdala comes to the rescue. It knows what to do when confronted with unexpected anger of this type!

Unfortunately, what it remembers is when you were 5-years old, crawled up on the kitchen counter had your hand in the cookie jar and your mother came around the corner and caught you in the act. One second you were slobbering in anticipation of a cookie and the next someone was yelling at you. Its immediate reaction is FREEZE!

Ummm, Houston, we have a problem . . .

All your nice, pleasant, friendly environment training is suddenly up against your nearly instinctual physical and emotional reaction.

This is why many martial artists fail when confronted with the real thing. It's not that they don't know how to react to the physical threat, but that they don't know how to respond to the emotional threat! You have to train yourself to handle both the physical problem and your emotional reactions! Without this ability, you're dog meat when confronted by the real thing.

The amygdala's conditioning takes place on a very, very deep level. It is trained around intense emotional stress. Unless you have lots of experience dealing with wild and unreasonable anger directed at you, that air-gulping sense of panic is still going to be your initial reaction! There can be lots of training layered over it, but until it gets to that level it won't be your amygdala's initial response.

If the amygdala doesn't have another preconditioned response, it's going to do what it knows to do. If that doesn't work, it's going to send a message back to the higher brain function for instructions because it doesn't know what else to do. In the meantime, you're standing there doing nothing while your higher brain tries to figure out what is the right response! Uh . . . er . . . fight or flight, maybe?

That is why that black belt sat down when her son's punk friend took a swing at her. She obviously had never had anyone swing at her in anger as an adult, especially someone she expected to intimidate. Her reactions weren't set up for that kind of thing That sort of stuff just doesn't happen to middle-aged mothers in small Western towns. Her poor amygdala was going bonkers! In the same vein, you can also see why Officer Adams handed back the gun. While he had trained and trained for that reaction, he hadn't trained himself on an emotional level when doing that move. His amygdala didn't register it as a threat, so his other training took over, and he handed the gun back.

Now the amygdala's reaction isn't set in concrete. It can be overcome and reprogrammed. The amygdala is always looking for bigger, better, faster ways of doing things to keep you alive and safe. But it has to be done on the same level as the original programming. And that kind of reprogramming only comes from actual experience or specifically tailored training.

Hopefully, you now see why I am such an advocate of scenario-based training. And why I go into conniption fits with people who think they can just waltz right out and translate martial arts training into the real thing.

[1]   *Anything Goes: Practical Karate for the Streets.* A good book. I highly recommend it if you want to research this topic further.

[2]   Unless you're really into reading technical scientific papers and articles. I must warn you, LeDoux's "Emotion and the Limbic System Concept" in *Concepts in Neuroscience 2,* 1992, nearly melted my brain. There are other important reasons to read Goleman's book. You'll get good information out of it about how people react and what to do about it.

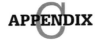

Combat Courses

*Begin by accepting the fact that all training
is based on the simulation of reality. The
operative word is simulation.*

—Bob Orlando
Martial Arts America

Below are the combat courses that I recommend. Just because a course isn't on the list doesn't mean it isn't good; it just means I haven't heard of it. What I do know, however, is that those listed here have solid, bulletproof track records. Most importantly, though, they deal with what goes on inside you as well as cracking heads.

Model Mugging/IMPACT
Check your local Yellow Pages under self-defense
for phone numbers
Web site:
http://www.bamm.org/chapters.html

Awakening the Warrior Within
Web site:
http://planetlink.lanminds.com/warrior/warrior.html
e-mail: awarrior@hooked.net

Rocky Mountain Combat Applications Training
PO Box 535, Lake George, CO 80827
Web site:
http//:members.aol.com/quinnp1/index.html
e-mail: quinnp1@aol.com

APPENDIX D

Books, Videos, and Other Stuff

....

Asked the experienced, not the learned.
—Arab Proverb

Throughout this book I've mentioned a whole load of other books and videos by other people. I firmly believe that no one person has a monopoly on the truth about crime, violence, or fighting. I have tried to give credit where credit is due, not just for concepts, but for terms that explain those concepts the best: Stevan Plinck's "Two Legged Milking Stool," Peyton Quinn's "Alien from Hell," Chris Caracci's "Orientation." None of these guys were saying anything that thousands of others haven't known over centuries, but they were the ones who came up with the terms that explain it best and easiest for Western minds.

Ever since I found a guy teaching my "Five Stages of Violent Crime" system without giving me credit (he claimed to have gotten it from a friend who got it from the FBI), I've been more and more aware of the tendency of people in this business to swipe something and teach it as their own. (It's amazing all the styles that suddenly had ancient and secret grappling techniques when Brazilian jujitsu hit the front pages.) This is the plagiarism side of "Not Invented Here." They can steal the good stuff and still look down their noses at everyone else. I don't believe in that. My contributions are mine, and other people deserve credit for theirs. Some of the people I mention here are my friends, others are people I have never met, but whose work I highly respect. Everything here is something that I consider street effective, real-life experienced, and lacking in wannabe B.S.

FROM PALADIN PRESS

Books

Hard Won Wisdom from the School of Hard Knocks: How to Avoid a Fight and Things to Do Whan You Can't or Don't Want To by Alain Burrese

Anything Goes: Practical Karate for the Streets by Loren W. Christensen

Close-Quarter Combat: A Soldier's Guide to Hand-to-Hand Fighting by Professor Leonard Holifield

Indonesian Fighting Fundamentals: The Brutal Arts of the Archipelago by Bob Orlando

Put 'Em Down, Take 'Em Out: Knife Fighting Techniques from Folsom Prison by Don Pentecost

Real Fighting: Adrenaline Stress Conditioning through Scenario-Based Training by Peyton Quinn

A Bouncer's Guide to Barroom Brawling: Dealing with the Sucker Puncher, Streetfighter, and Ambusher by Peyton Quinn

Championship Streetfighting: Boxing as a Martial Art by Ned Beaumont

1,001 Street Fighting Secrets: The Principles of Contemporary Fighting Arts by Sammy Franco

Videos

Practical Patrol Tactics for the 911 Officer with C.J. Caracci

Practical Hand-to-Hand Combat for the Police Officer with C.J. Caracci

Fighting Arts of Indonesia: Combat Secrets of Silat and Kuntao with Bob Orlando

Pukulan Pentjak Silat: The Devastating Fighting Art of Bukti Negara-Serak with Guru Stevan Plinck

MY STUFF FROM PALADIN

(Note: I first started writing these when I had just come off the street. While I seriously cleaned this book up, in all my other stuff my language is a little more . . . uh . . . colorful.)

Books

Cheap Shots, Ambushes, and Other Lessons: A Down and Dirty Book on Streetfighting and Survival

Knives, Knife Fighting, and Related Hassles: How to Survive a Real Knife Fight

Fists, Wits, and a Wicked Right: Surviving on the Wild Side of the Street

Pool Cues, Beer Bottles, and Baseball Bats: Animal's Guide to Improvised Weapons for Self-Defense and Survival

Floor Fighting: Stompings, Maimings, and Other Things to Avoid When a Fight Goes to the Ground

Street E&E: Evading, Escaping, and Other Ways to Save Your Ass When Things Get Ugly

A Professional's Guide to Ending Violence Quickly: How Bouncers, Bodyguards, and Other Security Professionals Handle Ugly Situations

Safe in the City: A Streetwise Guide to Avoid Being Robbed, Raped, Ripped Off, or Run Over (with Chris Pfouts)

Violence, Blunders, and Fractured Jaws: Advanced Awareness Techniques and Street Etiquette

Videos

Surviving a Street Knife Fight: Realistic Defensive Techniques (with Richard Dobson). Of the two knife videos, please get this one first, folks!

Winning a Street Knife Fight: Realistic Offensive Techniques (with Richard Dobson)

Down, But Not Out: Streetwise Tactics for Fighting on the Ground

Barroom Brawling: The Art of Staying Alive in Beer Joints, Biker Bars, and Other Fun Places (with Peyton Quinn)

Safe in the Street: How to Recognize and Avoid Violent Street Crime

BOOKS FROM OTHER PUBLISHERS

Not all of these are on self-defense, but they are important anyway.

Stressfire (Gunfighting for Police) by Massad Ayoob

Awakening the Warrior Within by Dawn Callan

Championship Fighting: Explosive Punching and Aggressive Defense by Jack Dempsey

Emotional Intelligence by Daniel Goleman

Filipino Martial Arts by Dan Inosanto

The Tao of Jeet Kun Do by Bruce Lee

Education of a Wandering Man by Louis L'Amour

Manwatching: A Field Guide to Human Behavior by Desmond Morris

Martial Arts America: A Western Approach to Eastern Arts by Bob Orlando

Inside the Criminal Mind by Stanton E. Samenow
Combat Strategy: Junsado, the Way of the Warrior
    by Hanho

    Oh yeah, I just realized I didn't mention it earli-
er, but I can be reached at:
    animalmac@aol.com
    http://www.diac.com/~dgordon